TAKE

CONTROL

OF YOUR

CANCER

Integrating the Best of Alternative and
Conventional Treatments

JAMES W. FORSYTHE, MD, HMD

 BENBELLA BOOKS, INC. | DALLAS, TEXAS

Copyright © 2012 James W. Forsythe, MD, HMD

All rights reserved. No part of this book may be used or reproduced in any manner whatsoever without written permission except in the case of brief quotations embodied in critical articles or reviews.

BenBella

BenBella Books, Inc.
10300 N. Central Expressway
Suite #400
Dallas, TX 75231
www.benbellabooks.com
Send feedback to feedback@benbellabooks.com

Printed in the United States of America

10 9 8 7 6 5 4 3 2 1

Library of Congress Cataloging-in-Publication Data is available for this title.

ISBN 978-1-936661-66-4

Editing by Erin Kelley
Copyediting by Shannon Kelly
Proofreading by Cape Cod Compositors, Inc.
Cover design by Allison Bard
Text design and composition by Neuwirth & Associates, Inc.
Printed by Berryville Graphics

Distributed by Perseus Distribution
perseusdistribution.com

To place orders through Perseus Distribution:
Tel: 800-343-4499
Fax: 800-351-5073
E-mail: orderentry@perscusbooks.com

Significant discounts for bulk sales are available. Please contact Glenn Yeffeth at glenn@benbellabooks.com or 214-750-3628.

CONTENTS

PART 1

PART 2

To my loving wife, Earlene, without whom I would not have been driven to write this exposé. To my five children—Marc, Michele, Lisa, Pompeo, and Sarah—and our blessed ten grandchildren—Kiley, Clayton, Teson, Previn, Sebastian, Luke, Ryker, Liam, Antonio, and Julia.

And most of all, to the more than 10,000 cancer patients I have treated throughout the world during the past forty years. It has been my goal and my passion to make their lives with cancer more bearable, while respecting their body's pillars of strength with emphasis on their diet, nutrition, and immune system integrity.

Thank you to all of these patients, from whom I have learned something valuable in my practice of integrative oncology to carry forward. This book is dedicated to you.

It is a rare occurrence when an insider in the field of medical oncology dares to speak out against the forces of the Federal Drug Administration (FDA), Big Pharmaceutical, and the conventional oncology establishment in order to bring reason to an area of medicine that has essentially lost the forty-year-old "war on cancer," and which has spent more than $100 billion of taxpayer money in the process.

But Dr. James W. Forsythe is that insider! He is multicredentialed and has impeccable education and certification credentials. His pedigree includes more than sixteen years of post-high-school training: a BA from the University of California at Berkeley, an MD from the University of California at San Francisco, a US Army internship and residency in pathology, an internal medicine residency in San Francisco, an oncology fellowship at the University of California at San Francisco, and a certification in homeopathy in Nevada.

If that was not enough, Dr. Forsythe is also a certified medical director of nursing homes, a former director of five clinical laboratories, and is board-eligible in gerontology and anti-aging medicine. His military career includes twenty-six years of service in the US Army and Reserves and in the National Guard, with commendation medals from his duty in Vietnam and his service as the state surgeon for the Nevada Army National Guard, where he retired as a full colonel.

Unlike doctors who practice conventional oncology, Dr. Forsythe reviews the etiologies of cancer, which number more than three dozen. He then gives you an honest appraisal of what to expect from standard chemotherapy protocols. He also outlines the most common myths of conventional cancer treatments—of great importance to cancer patients.

This book is a must-read for cancer patients, for their families and friends, and for medical students who are often brainwashed by medical school curricula, which teaches that Big Pharma has the only solution to Stage IV cancer treatments.

In the literature of Big Pharma itself, in both the United States and Australia, five-year chemotherapy results for Stage IV adult cancers yields a disheartening 2.1% to 2.3% survival rate—nothing more needs to be said.

Dr. Forsythe and I think alike on these matters, and I would wholeheartedly recommend reading this exposé!

Dr. Burton Goldberg
Author of *Alternative Medicine:*
The Definitive Guide (2nd edition)

WHY I ABANDONED CONVENTIONAL ONCOLOGY

At least once in every cancer specialist's career, a near-death patient appears who inexplicably undergoes a profound healing transformation, resulting in the attending physician becoming haunted by the mystery of what happened and why. For me, that first special patient was a middle-aged woman I had been treating for metastic melanoma to the liver in the early 1980s.

Christine (name changed) had melanoma that had metastasized into several tumors on her liver. She was undergoing conventional chemotherapy when something strange happened; while putting on her boots one day, she was bitten on the leg by a brown recluse spider. Her leg swelled up tremendously, and she had to go to the hospital for treatment. About three weeks after this spider bite, we performed an ultrasound on her and discovered something that shocked the entire medical team—the liver tumors were gone. It seemed as though the spider venom had jump-started Christine's immune systems and vanquished the cancer; it was the only new agent introduced into her body.

Oncologists usually dismiss any anecdotes about miraculous remissions and cancer cures, even though most of them have encountered cases of remission they can't explain. Not only do conventionally trained cancer specialists not want to hear about cases such as Christine's, they are hostile toward any physician (like me) who takes an interest in these anecdotes.

Christine's remarkable recovery intrigued me. Her experience seemed to indicate that the human immune system can be provoked into successfully treating cancer, even serious cases of the disease like Christine's. I began to consider whether this could be done more readily using other substances without resorting to something as strong and as unpredictable as spider venom.

All of my oncology colleagues in the eighties had a conventional outlook toward cancer treatment. Their approach was always to use full-dose chemotherapy and never deviate from accepted protocols. We knew that chemo was killing good cells, but we just hoped it was killing enough bad cells too. There were fewer than twenty drugs being used in those early days of oncology and they had devastating side effects. All of the patients became horribly sick from the treatment and most of them relapsed within a few years.

When I entered the field of oncology medicine in the early 1970s at the University of California at San Francisco, it was a relatively new subspecialty of internal medicine. President Richard Nixon had declared the federal War on Cancer, and there was a lot of hope that with this huge influx of funding for cancer research, we might soon find a cure, or at the very least develop some treatments that extended the life spans of cancer patients.

My entry into the cancer field occurred the first year that the boards were offered for this certification, and I joined a class of what later turned out to contain the "rock stars" of oncology. Included in this group were Sydney Salmon, MD; David Golde, MD; Mick Haskell, MD; and David Albers, MD. All of these physicians would head up programs at various universities across the country and become extremely important figures in the field of cancer treatment.

It was during my training at UC San Francisco that I discovered how arbitrary the cancer treatment protocols we were learning had already become. Someone higher up in the field would get an idea that we should prescribe a particular drug twice a week for this or that cancer and it should be the standard dose. Many times there was no scientific evidence behind what they were saying. Because we were trainees, we had to follow their exact protocol, whether it was evidence based or not.

Some drugs came in such a high dose that every single patient who was prescribed the drug had to have the dose lowered. Every recommendation was arbitrary, and it put our patients on the losing end of a vicious trial and error. And despite the lack of evidence, these physicians and administrators were declaring the protocol to be an exact science, a sort of gold standard for medical practice. The obvious shortcomings bothered me a lot.

When I attended oncology conventions there would be an exercise in which a cancer case would be presented and everyone would vote on how they would treat that particular case. There was never a consensus about treatment. Of the specialists present, 60% might say one type of drug should be used, while 40% voted otherwise. I would think to myself, "How can this be?" These physicians were all oncologists. They should have been on the same page. But they never were; unfortunately for cancer patients, they still aren't.

More than 100 cancer drugs are out there today (some in use without FDA approval), and there is no consensus on which drugs to use, what doses to use, how long to give them, or which types of cancer respond best to those drugs. All of these decisions are made arbitrarily, turning the patients into virtual guinea pigs.

MY APPROACH TO TREATMENT EVOLVES

The biggest epiphany for me following Christine's spider-bite-induced cancer remission came after consulting the cancer survival rates. Five years after being diagnosed with cancer, only 2% of Stage IV cancer patients were still alive, after being subjected to repeated rounds of slash-and-burn treatment.

Confirmation of my observations later came in an article written in the *Journal of Oncology* in 2004 that noted how "in a large retrospective study, the overall survival rate for patients with Stage IV cancer receiving chemotherapy was only 2.1% in the United States, and in a similar study done in Australia showed only a 2.3% survival rate."

This finding showed me that the over-treatment approach and the treatment protocols using so many toxins constituted a failing strategy. Even if you were lucky enough to be one of those two out of a hundred who survived, you would probably have chemo brain symptoms, you might have heart and liver problems, and you would probably experience constant pain and the loss of feeling in your feet and toes. These were just accepted side effects.

Oncologists didn't want to think about this dismal 2% survival rate after five years. Understandably, they didn't want to acknowledge that they were doing any harm to their patients. They got upset when they learned that someone like me was deviating from the standard protocol and using much lower doses of these drugs with better results. Most specialists simply refuse to believe that we can get much better results by using much lower doses, because to someone who is used to treating illnesses with medication, it seems like "more" and "stronger" must always be better.

What further disturbed me was the astounding escalation in patient treatment costs, especially when they were being directed to use toxic or ineffective cancer drugs following surgery. These high-dose drugs are expensive and often problematic. One lung cancer drug was on the market for almost five years and cost patients $25,000 a year, based on them taking one pill a day, yet studies found the drug to be no more effective than if the patients had taken a placebo sugar pill every day. This amounted to a royal fleecing of people who had been rendered vulnerable and fearful by the prospect of a painful death.

I finally broke my ties with the standard oncology practices and changed my cancer treatment practice in Reno, Nevada to Integrative Oncology. In the early '70s there were no other certified oncologists in northern Nevada, and only two in Las Vegas. During the next few years, I helped to develop cancer wards at Reno's two major facilities: St. Mary's Hospital and Washoe Medical Center. I often had more than forty patients a day under my care. After ten years of medical practice in Reno, my disenchantment with the results of standard treatments reached its zenith.

Those individuals who were lucky enough to survive Stage IV cancers often suffered from many of the symptoms of toxic chemotherapy. These included everything from chemo brain syndrome to peripheral neuropathies (nerve damage), cardiomyopathy (heart muscle disease), liver failure, kidney failure, hearing problems, and severe bone marrow depressions requiring repeated transfusions of red cells and platelets.

The quality of their lives, even though they may have survived cancer, was oftentimes dismal and I found myself wondering if it survival was worth the price. There was a morbid saying at some of our oncology meetings: "We cured the cancer, but the patient died."

Gradually, I began to embrace some alternatives to conventional treatment. In Reno I had been receiving cancer referrals from local naturopaths and homeopaths and I became curious about their use of vitamin and mineral supplements, which sometimes seemed to show good results. So I started going to their meetings and talking with them, curious about how I could incorporate what they did into my oncology practice.

The concept of homeopathy appealed to me because it involves provoking the immune system into action using tiny doses of substances, much as Christine's immune system had been jump-started by spider venom. I started working with a homeopathy clinic in Reno that was seeing forty to fifty patients a day. I would arrive there after my regular office hours and see two or three cancer patients from five to seven p.m., letting them know what I would do conventionally, since that's the kind of treatment I knew how to do at the time. I ended up being so impressed with the results I was seeing that I got my own degree in homeopathy, becoming board certified in Nevada in 1996.

Homeopathy has been around for several hundred years and teaches that small doses can stimulate immune reactions in the body, triggering the immune system to fight whatever ailment afflicts the patient. In principle, this is the same idea that is the basis for vaccines, which inject a small dose of the disease into the bloodstream, in order to stimulate your immune system into creating antibodies.

Rather than become a classic homeopathic practitioner and completely abandon my medical education, I decided instead to integrate homeopathic principles into my oncology practice. I began to create a medical niche that pushed the treatment envelope—in a manner that was both safe and within the confines of the law—by combining natural therapy with conventional oncology to provide maximum benefit to my patients.

When some of my medical colleagues began to realize that I was thinking outside the conventional box about cancer treatment, I lost some referrals and friendships. I was no longer welcome at meetings attended by certain other oncologists. They labeled my method a pseudo-science, something that isn't evidence based. Because they didn't learn about it in medical school, they considered it mere quackery. The bottom line is that they simply didn't—and many still don't—have the courage to deviate from Big Pharma's indoctrination and drug-obsessed dogma.

Under the prevailing dogma, if you receive a heavy dose of chemo and you die after your first treatment, it's considered okay because the oncologist did everything by the book. The oncologist has no liability as a result. I know from firsthand experience that at the Kaiser hospitals, which are operated by the Veterans Health Administration hospitals, oncologists and physicians aren't allowed to talk about supplements or diet as part of cancer treatment. Their protocol is chemotherapy, using exact doses by the book, and when you get nausea or other side effects, they give you another drug for that and expect you to be content with the consequences.

WHAT AN INTEGRATIVE ONCOLOGIST DOES DIFFERENTLY

Chemosensitivity testing is an important first step that I use in treatment, which conventional oncologists typically don't use. It's a test we send to a European lab or one in Texas, to break down cancer genes and biomarkers so we know exactly which drugs and supplements to give a patient to have the most positive effect on their particular type of cancer.

I foresee chemosensitivity testing becoming a standard procedure in every oncologist's office. But it isn't now, not until the US Food and Drug Administration gives its approval, and that unconscionable delay is causing cancer patients needless pain and suffering when they receive chemotherapy drugs in doses that they don't need, or when they're given drugs that don't work effectively for the type of cancer they have.

If I am giving you chemo that isn't working, then I am just giving you a poison. It's a waste of your time, your money, and your immune system's precious resources. Meanwhile, your cancer is left to continue its deadly growth.

These chemosensitivity tests do work. I have seen their value firsthand, countless times, with patients on whom conventional oncologists had given up.

For a patient to choose an alternative cancer therapy may require the courage to resist pressures of friends, family, and physicians. I have noticed that patients who dare to mention to their oncologist their interest in pursuing an alternative therapy are given mostly negative responses, or brushed off with, "I didn't learn that in medical school; it's not evidence-based medicine."

Some conventionally trained oncologists even tell patients that they will refuse to treat them if they pursue any alternative treatments. That can be intimidating to patients. I also hear patients complain that their oncologist never talked about diet, nutrition, or supplements, brushing the subjects off as unimportant. The oncologist might also say that the supplements would interfere with chemotherapy.

An integrative oncologist always asks questions to help identify what caused the cancer in the first place. Though this seems like common sense, it is rare for a conventional oncologist to do this. Did the patient grow up on a farm around lots of pesticides and insecticides? Does the patient have a mouth full of dental metals? Have chemical exposures on the job played a role? Do they have an underlying viral condition, such as hepatitis B or C, that's associated with liver cancer? What kind of diet does the patient have?

This is all very important to know in order to help prevent a recurrence of the cancer. An integrative oncologist like myself wants to know all of this information to prevent the cancer from recurring. Allergy testing, hair analysis, and other tests can also help to pinpoint possible triggers for the cancer.

In order for integrative oncology to be accepted by conventional oncologists, I decided that clinical, outcome-based studies had to be conducted on natural products offered to the patients, either alone or in addition to chemotherapy in their traditional form by protocol, or in modified forms such as fractionated dosing or dosing with insulin potentiation. In this way we could dispel the notion that integrative oncology wasn't evidence-based medicine.

To assemble such evidence, I crafted and performed studies on Paw Paw Cell Reg for health-supplement manufacturer Nature's Sunshine, involving more than 100 patients, and on Poly-MVA for Garnett McKeen Laboratories, a study that accrued more than 225 patients. In fact, the FDA subpoenaed my Poly-MVA studies and has reviewed my current Forsythe Immune Therapy study.

The Forsythe Immune Therapy contains, in part, a homeopathic glyco-benzaldehyde compound that interferes with the fermentation of sugar in the cancer cell, thus depriving the cancer of its main source of nutrition. The current study of Forsythe Immune Therapy containing the glyco-benzaldehyde homeopathic remedy has produced response rates of 45% in more than 500 patients with Stage IV cancers at five years' duration. Our individual cancer results are running in the 0 – 100% positive response range, with best responders being in breast, prostate, lung, and lymphoma cancers. An overall response rate of 46% has been achieved in this study, results that are superior to any known statistics compiled by the conventional allopathic literature.

During my four decades of practice in Northern Nevada, I have overseen more than 200,000 patient visits. I always offer my cancer patients three standard options: first is conventional chemotherapy alone, second is conventional chemotherapy along with complementary therapy, and third is complementary therapy alone. You will find all of these options described in this book.

✳

If you or someone you know and love has been diagnosed with cancer, you deserve access to all of the possibly effective treatment options that can reduce suffering and save a life. If you are open to expanding your range of treatment therapies, or in researching them on behalf of someone else in need, this book was written with you in mind.

1

YOUR

CONVENTIONAL

CANCER

TREATMENT

OPTION

CHAPTER ONE

YOUR WARNING SIGNS OF CANCER

What should you look for to detect the warning signs or symptoms of cancer? Let's start with the most obvious.

Skin is the most common site of all cancers and these may show up as a lesion or growth that you notice on your face, extremities, or trunk, arising unexpectedly.

These are the questions that you should start asking yourself: Does the lesion continue to grow, or does it ulcerate? Is it tender? Does it bleed? Does it have a black or dark color, or various shades of brown? Is your skin taking on a yellow cast? Are the whites of your eyes more yellow than white? Are there growing nodules or lumps just under the surface of the skin that have never been noticed before, and have they been growing larger over a short period of time? Unfortunately, there is no one symptom that can indicate whether or not you have cancer, but if you start noticing any of these symptoms suddenly, or multiple symptoms that seem connected, it's time to contact a doctor.

Other symptoms to watch for:

In your neck, axillae (armpits), and groin regions, are your glands and lymph nodes enlarging but non-tender?

Are you having unexplained low-grade fevers or night sweats?

Is your skin itchy for no apparent reason?

Do you have a persistent, red, or blotchy rash that is not painful to the touch and not related to an allergic contact?

In general, are you losing weight without dieting? Is your appetite poor? Is your energy level reduced?

Are there any sores in your mouth or on your tongue that do not heal within a two-week period, and for which there is no obvious cause?

Is your swallowing impaired? Does food get "hung up" or seem to not go completely through into the stomach?

Are you having persistent nausea, vomiting, or diarrhea without explanation?

Do you have unexplained bleeding from any orifice including the mouth, nose, anus, vagina, or urethra?

Are you having any unexplained pains in the head, neck, chest, abdomen, back, or extremities, without any history of trauma or infection?

Do you experience the sudden onset of increasing shortness of breath, prolonged cough, spitting up of blood, or pleurisy?

Are there any changes in your bowel movements? These would include changes in the color of your stool to black, maroon, silver, or tan. Do your stools float in the bowl? Do your stools look flattened in shape, or pencil-like?

Is there any pain or bleeding with intercourse? Have you had postmenopausal bleeding or bleeding between menstrual cycles? Is your abdominal waist size enlarging without weight gain? Do you look four to five months pregnant?

Are your breasts swollen or tender? Is there any nipple discharge or bleeding? Do you feel any discrete lumps or nodules in any portion of your breasts or axillary areas that you've never noticed before? Are your breasts noticeably different sizes, without any reasonable explanation?

Are there any unexplained swellings or asymmetry of either testicle, not related to trauma or infection? Is there any abnormal discharge from your urethra or penis?

Is there any abrupt change in your mental functioning, motor or sensory loss, or problems with coordination or balance? Have you experienced any type of mild or major seizures, including blackouts, memory lapses, or any unexplained mood changes?

When any of these disturbing signs or symptoms appear, persist, or worsen over time, it is imperative that a prompt and thorough medical evaluation be done to establish a correct diagnosis!

A renowned, now deceased, Canadian physician, William Osler, once said that the most important factor in achieving a proper treatment is a correct diagnosis, a correct diagnosis, and a correct diagnosis!

Make an appointment as soon as possible and clearly describe your symptoms to your primary care medical doctor, who may be a family physician, an internist, or even a gynecolo-gist, depending on where your symptoms are located. Be the "squeaky wheel" and make sure that your physician, physician's assistant, or advanced nurse practitioner takes your concerns seriously and orders the appropriate tests. Also, make sure that a complete examination, including a rectal examination and a pelvic examination, is performed, as well as a complete neuro-logical examination.

GET THOROUGHLY TESTED

Screening laboratory tests most commonly include—at the very least—a complete blood count (CBC), a comprehensive meta-bolic panel, and a urinalysis. More complete testing will often include a hormonal profile, a vitamin D3 level, an immune competency profile, including a natural killer cell (NKC) assay, and specific tumor marker testing for cancers related to defini-tive organs such as breast, lung, prostate, liver, etc.

A hair analysis for toxic metals is advisable, but this proce-dure is usually done only by physicians practicing integrative or alternative medicine.

Keep in mind that not all cancers will present with blood or urine tumor markers. Those that don't show such markers include brain cancers, head and neck cancers, uterine and cer-vical cancers, and sarcomas and kidney cancers.

Once the testing has been completed and a suspicion is raised by the combination of a finding on your physical exami-nation, laboratory studies, urinalysis, immune panel, or tumor markers, it is customary for the medical practitioner to call the patient in for a follow-up consultation and to give their opinion of the possible diagnoses, either one or many. When a tumor marker test is done, a doctor is looking for protein fragments that arise from cancer. These are foreign to the body, and show up as an antigen. A higher count relates to more cancer cells in the body.

It is important to realize that the laboratory workup already may have made the diagnosis without a further biopsy or other invasive test being ordered. An example of this would be the finding on a complete blood count (CBC) of either an acute or chronic leukemia, which may be obvious simply by looking at the findings on the CBC.

Another example would be a high tumor marker, such as the combination of a high CA-125 coupled with the finding of a mass on pelvic examination, denoting an ovarian cancer in the lower quadrants of the abdomen on physical examination. CA-125 is a specific tumor marker used primarily to diagnose ovarian cancer, but can also be present in an elevated state for those who have lung or uterine cancer.

GET A BIOPSY

Despite these exceptions, it is the *sine qua non*, or absolute necessity, that a tissue biopsy be obtained in order to follow through and design the appropriate therapeutic approach.

Rarely is this ironclad rule in medicine violated. Exceptions are in cases of a deep-seated brain tumor or internal cancers in a patient for whom invasive surgical biopsy has been deemed an unacceptable risk. In every other instance a tissue diagnosis is mandatory!

The biopsy may be as simple as a skin, a lymph node, or a

bone marrow biopsy done as an outpatient or in a same-day surgical center.

More complex biopsies include needle biopsies of the lung, liver, or kidney, possibly associated with endoscopy procedures either in the head/neck areas, larynx, trachea, bronchial tubes, esophagus, stomach, duodenum, or colon. Even more complex biopsies would include those done under anesthesia in the mediastinum (structures in the thorax), chest cavities, peritoneal cavities, brain tissues, or testes.

Oftentimes a frozen section is done on the more complex biopsies with a pathologist either present in the operating room or standing by in the laboratory to tell the surgeon if the tissue submitted is adequate enough to make a solid pathologic diagnosis.

AN ONCOLOGIST STEPS IN

Once a specific diagnosis is made of a cancer, and it is identified as being specific to a definite organ site, anatomical site, or blood-forming tissue, the next step for the primary care physician or surgeon is to refer the patient to a medical oncologist. The oncologist's job is to determine, through the laboratory or radiology studies, if the disease is that of the primary site of origin or whether the cancer has spread locally or has travelled to distant sites such as the lung, liver, bones, or brain tissues. As many as 5% of biopsies arrive at a diagnosis of "cancer at an unknown primary site," so-called CUP.

Early regional spread may occur in nearby lymph nodal sites, and is often determined by the pathologist under gross or microscopic inspection of the submitted surgical tissues. For instance, in breast cancer, any spread to same-side lymph nodes renders the patient at that point with at least a Stage II designation. In cases of more distant nodal spread involving the lymph nodes in nearby areas such as the area surrounding the clavicles, a Stage III diagnosis is the minimum staging classification.

It would then customarily fall upon the shoulders of the oncologist to perform a metastatic survey to determine if any distant metastases exist. Metastases are cancers that have spread via direct invasion of the blood or lymph fluid and migrated to a site other than where it originated. This survey includes chest X-rays, ultrasounds, CAT scans, and at the very most, PET scans of the body, to determine if in fact distant spread has occurred.

The simplest and least invasive of these procedures, at a minimum, would include a chest X-ray, a liver ultrasound, and a nuclear medicine bone scan.

An intermediate level of testing would include CAT scans or MRI scanning. CAT scanning is preferred on brain tissues and on the chest and abdominal areas, whereas MRI scanning is performed on extremities and soft tissue areas, and in some cases also on brain tissues where there are no internal movements.

The "gold standard" and most invasive testing is that of the PET scan, which by radiological standards delivers as much radiation to the recipient as the entire combination of a head, chest, abdomen, pelvis, and bone scan combined. Because of the radiation levels involved, it is not recommended that this scan be done more than once a year, and even less so if possible.

The PET scan is based upon the fact that cancer cells, out of necessity, rely upon simple sugars for their main source of nutrition. The scan itself uses a radio-tagged sugar molecule to essentially "light up" cancer anywhere in the body, except in the brain tissues, which also rely upon sugar as a main source of energy.

Incidentally, the PET scan is not definitive by any means. A cancer deposit or metastasis must reach a diameter between 5.0 and 10.0 mm. before it can even be detected on a PET scan. Therefore, a sizeable amount of cancer could be present in the body and not be detected at all on PET scanning.

After enumerating all of your symptoms, do not allow your doctor to over-test your body with excessive amounts of radiation including excessive CAT scans or PET scans, which can often make your condition worse by weakening your immune system. Keep in mind that a CAT scan is tantamount to as many as 100 simple chest X-rays.

CHAPTER TWO

IF YOU ARE DIAGNOSED WITH CANCER

Once the cancer verdict is given, it's certainly understandable that the cancer patient might become overwhelmed with a range of emotions.

Here are examples of the many reactions that I have personally witnessed from my own cancer patients in four decades of practicing medical oncology. Once the word "cancer" has been mentioned they feel blinded and deafened by the word itself. Patients have often described having the feeling of a deer in the headlights who is watching a speeding car come at them head-on and not being able to move. They often feel numb and immobile, as if their thought processes are on hold.

The wide variety of emotions patients experience includes denial, shock and disbelief, anxiety and confusion, fear and self-pity, and anger and hopelessness. Many people immediately feel the loss of not being able to live out the happiness of their marriage or to see their children grow, graduate, marry, and have grandchildren.

Some patients erupt with a flood of questions. A common one is, "How long do I have, Doc?" The next question is usually, "What will this treatment do to me? What toxicities will I have to endure?" Another common question that oncologists hear is, "How will you know when I am cured?"

Cancer patients are often the easiest patients for a physician to work with because they have been rendered compliant by fear and anxiety. They normally cooperate with the oncologist because they are afraid of dying. They rarely think about doing any independent research to help clarify their options; instead, they just rely on their physician to tell them what to do.

DON'T BE RUSHED INTO A DECISION

A physician may simply tell the patient to show up in the operating room or the radiation suite the following Monday. Oftentimes a practitioner will, intentionally or not, scare the patient into making a treatment decision rapidly, without allowing them to do any research on their own about other possible treatments or therapies.

Among the things that every cancer patient should remember is that by the time their cancer has been detected, it has probably been growing in their body for months or years. Therefore, an immediate decision regarding treatment therapy isn't normally necessary because one more day or one more week, or even one more month, may not make a difference in their survival.

In rare cases, the doctor will tell a patient that the cancer is too far advanced to do any treatment whatsoever. In cases like this the patient should simply thank their doctor and leave. Go seek a second or third opinion, especially an alternative medicine opinion, because the primary doctor has already given up and has no intention of providing anything other than hospice care.

Remember, if an oncologist starts talking about hospice care and "getting your affairs in order," that oncologist has given up on you, something that I believe no doctor should ever do.

In my practice, I always try to err on the side of optimism with patients. I never give them a prognosis or a time frame for survival. I've had patients come to me saying their doctors had told them not to start a new novel or start watching a new soap opera because they wouldn't be alive long enough to see the ending. I think it's cruel to treat a patient with a terminal illness this way. I am flabbergasted that any physician would try to play God by predicting the end of a patient's life. When a case is considered terminal, doctors will often make these cruel remarks or suggest hospice care instead of any treatment options. Before a patient accepts their doctor's recommendation for hospice care, there are a few things they should know.

✶

Five years ago, a patient might be in a hospice for six months. With hospice care today it may be twenty-four to forty-eight hours because the morphine is being turned up hourly, and as the morphine goes up, respiration goes down. So a patient going into hospice is usually dead within seventy-two hours because they no longer have any active chemo, radiation, or treatment of any sort other than morphine to relieve pain.

Which is better? Some would say it's better to get a "terminal" life over fast.

It bothers me that when a patient goes into hospice, the insurance company provides only a finite amount of money. So the faster a patient dies, the more money the insurance company saves. Sometimes doctors are influenced by this insurance company incentive to get patients into hospice sooner rather than later just to save the company money.

In larger community hospitals, hospitals that are run by the Veterans Health Administration, university centers, and major cancer centers, difficult cancer cases are often presented to a standing tumor board of interested physicians. These boards, as a rule, are run by the pathology department and always include the involved surgeon or surgeons, the pathologist, the oncologist, the radiologist, and the referring primary care physician and any other interested staff physicians.

While there is always hope for a unanimous opinion as to the proper course of treatment, most often there is no consensus of opinion and it is left up to the referring physician or oncologist to make the final treatment decision. (In my experience, lack of consensus is the norm. At the hundreds of cancer conferences I've attended over thirty years, where several hundred oncologists vote on treatment recommendations—whether for difficult or seemingly routine cases—100% consensus is rarely achieved. This has continued to surprised me, and only further disproves the existence of hard-and-fast evidence-based therapies upon which all oncologists agree.)

After the tumor board deliberation, or simply at the stage of the lone oncologist preparing a treatment protocol, it is time for the patient and the patient's family to agree or disagree to proceed with the recommended treatment plan. This is probably the most difficult decision any patient has ever had to make.

EMPOWER YOURSELF WITH RESEARCH

As soon as the diagnosis comes in, take control of your own health and empower yourself through learning and knowledge. Doing so could very well save your life.

Don't rush into surgery or radiation without knowing all of the possible complications, both short- and long-term. For example, a radical prostate removal is not a simple procedure. A fifty-year-old man whose prostate has been removed will face an 80% chance of erectile dysfunction for the remaining twenty or thirty years of his life. On top of that, sometimes other side effects appear, like bladder problems, pain from the procedure, risks associated with anesthesia in surgery, and hospital-borne infections. Complications can occur. All of this needs to be factored into the equation when considering conventional approaches to treatment.

There are other important considerations that are rarely addressed by conventional oncologists. You should know the cancer's specific nutritional requirements, its need for simple sugars, its need for an acidic environment, its need for a low-oxygen environment, and the fact that cancer cells are low energy systems, meaning they only produce 5% of the cellular energy as a normal cell produces. A cancer cell's major mission is to kill its host.

Something else to consider is that a cancer cell's growth is variable. Many cancers are extremely slow-growing. Other cancer cells may lie dormant for years, even decades. The end result, however, remains the same—the cancer's primary mission is to end your life, and in so doing, it ends its own life. It is basically a suicide bomber.

The primary mission for the patient going forward from the point of diagnosis should be to look for other options, to seek a second opinion, especially an opinion from a physician practicing integrative or alternative medicine.

CHAPTER THREE

TREATMENTS THEY WILL OFFER YOU

Once all of the information generated by testing has been presented to you, the conventional oncologist typically schedules another appointment and discusses the most acceptable protocol for treatment, based on what has been established by the National Cancer Institute.

These protocols provide a road map of sorts for treating a patient's specific histology, pathologic grade, tumor markers, and hormonal status, if this is appropriate. These protocols often include the stage of the disease, as well as the age and performance status of the patient, and lists of approved drugs by Medicare and Medicaid. Radiation therapy or the use of various types of radiation, including external beam, radioactive seed therapy, proton beam therapy, or CyberKnife radiology therapy—which is given before, during, or after chemotherapy—is also often included in these protocols.

As part of the general therapeutic program, lists of hormonal options and targeted therapy options may be offered for cancers where these treatments are appropriate.

To add to the barrage of information that's being thrown at the patient, conventional oncologists now use various Internet prognosticating programs to determine outcome percentages based on whether certain protocols are followed or not followed. These programs make the conventional oncologist look like he or she is basing his or her decision strictly on evidence-based medicine. The intention is to give the patient confidence that the oncologist knows what he or she is doing. These programs take into consideration the histology (the physical makeup) of the tumor, the grade (degree of abnormality) of the tumor, the stage (spread and advancement) of the cancer, and hormonal markers (which hormones are included in the tumor), including genetic markers, and attempt to provide the patient with the risks and rewards for following specific recommended guidelines. Unfortunately, these programs are often faulty and inaccurate.

Unbeknownst to the patient, who is often unsophisticated in the medical arena, the conventional oncologist cannot and does not know for sure whether any of the treatments being proposed will work for that specific patient's cancer. The reason for this is that the oncologist is basing all recommendations upon the latest clinical studies, none of which ever reveal a 100% response rate. In most cases, the oncologist does not inform the patient that there is a possibility that none of these therapies could work for his or her specific cancer.

SLASH, BURN, AND POISON

After the treatment details have been discussed with you by your oncologist or surgeon, the full force of conventional oncology kicks into overdrive in the form of surgery, radiation therapy, and chemotherapy, either singly, doubly or in triplicate.

We practitioners in alternative or integrative medicine refer to these conventional options as "slash, burn, and poison."

Rarely, if ever, does any meaningful discussion of secondary options take place evaluating diet, nutrition, alkalinization, bio-oxidative therapies, or supplements. In fact, if the patient (after doing some research) inquires about these lines of treatment, he or she is generally dismissed by the physician with a stern look and a categorical statement of negativity, such as: "They are useless. They will do you no good! There is no evidence-based science behind any of these options." And finally, the oncologist might even issue an ultimatum: "If you choose to use anything but conventional therapy, you will have to find another oncologist!"

These statements tell the patient that the physician is in charge and has closed his or her mind to all alternative therapies. At this point, the patient knows that seeking a second opinion, especially an alternative medicine opinion, had better be done covertly or else a new oncologist must be found.

The usual sequence of treatments depends on the stage of the tumor more than any other single factor. Here is what you can expect:

Lung Cancers: In early-stage disease, the treatment may be simply surgery, with or without follow-up radiation therapy.

In Stage IV disease, the desired conventional treatment may consist of surgery followed by chemotherapy, or chemotherapy alone.

Breast Cancers: In early-stage breast cancer, conventional treatment is usually surgery in the form of a simple lumpectomy or a more extensive modified radical mastectomy. In Stage II breast cancer, it would be commonplace to have surgery first, followed by chemotherapy and then by radiation therapy. The use of radiation therapy after these two modalities is in question as no physician at this point really knows what they are treating since there is no way to measure if there is in fact any residual disease. In Stage IV breast cancer, surgery and radiation therapy may be bypassed completely for long-term chemotherapy alone or with additional hormonal, targeted, and/or Herceptin treatments.

Colorectal Cancers: In early-stage disease, chemotherapy and radiation therapy are often used first, and this is called neo-adjuvant therapy. Afterwards, if the chemotherapy and radiation don't work, definitive surgery would be the third-place treatment procedure. In advanced colorectal cancers, surgery may be necessary first, in order to avoid bowel obstruction from the growing tumor, especially if it is in the left colon. This would then be followed with chemotherapy, with or without some form of targeted therapy.

Prostate Cancers: In early-stage prostate cancers, especially in a man between forty and sixty years old, radical surgery or radiation therapy in the form of external beam, brachytherapy, or proton beam therapy is usually proposed. For

Stage IV prostate cancers, surgery and radiation therapy are generally avoided in favor of hormonal therapy; only if the patient becomes hormonally resistant will chemotherapy be offered. The term "radical surgery" in regard to prostate cancer many times scares patients toward either radiation or hormonal therapies, since patients are terrified of losing whole internal organs.

Brain Cancers: In primary brain cancers (meaning cancers that started in the brain), the standard sequence of treatment would be surgery in the form of debulking the primary tumor site, followed by radiation therapy—either localized or whole-brain radiation therapy—and then chemotherapy. Occasionally targeted therapy is done in combination. Some deep-seated or strategically placed central nervous system tumors may be impossible to biopsy and, therefore, radiation therapy followed by chemotherapy are used without any pathologic diagnosis. The same sequence may occur in inoperable pancreatic tumors.

Kidney Cancers: In Stage IV kidney cancers, the kidney may still be removed as an initial procedure, as this cancer is one of the rare cancers that when the primary, or mother, tumor is removed, the secondary (daughter) tumors may spontaneously subside or disappear, even without the radiation or chemotherapy follow-up.

Cervical or Uterine Cancers: Following a positive biopsy by a gynecologist, patients with early-stage disease often undergo radiation therapy followed by surgery. If metastases are present at the time of surgery, follow-up chemotherapy is then generally recommended. In Stage IV uterine or cervical cancers, chemotherapy alone is the treatment of choice.

TAKE CONTROL OF YOUR LIFE

This is the point where the patient must take full control of his or her destiny. Although the conventional oncologist is well-meaning and feels he or she is using his or her skills and knowledge to design the best protocol for the patient based upon the latest publicized clinical studies, the patient's cancer is not being treated specifically, nor is the whole patient being treated.

Missing from the protocol of radiation or chemotherapy alone are the most important physiological and biochemical properties of the growing cancer and the consideration of various important factors, including proper diet and supplements, acid-based balancing, bio-oxidative factors, and the underlying energetics of the cancer cell itself.

Also absent from conventional protocols is genetic chemosensitivity testing on the patient's whole blood, an absolutely essential procedure that can precisely pinpoint the specific drugs necessary to treat the patient's cancer. This testing is foreign to almost all conventional oncologists in the United States, but is commonly employed by oncologists in Europe—especially at the high-tech laboratories in Germany and Greece—and Asia.

For the integrative oncologist, this genetic testing is as important for determining the proper drugs to prescribe as it is for determining which supplements, hormones, and targeted therapies will work best against the patient's specific cancer cells. This information is vital and serves as a blueprint for identifying the best drugs and the best supplements for each particular patient. Without using these modalities (which tell which drugs and supplements will be effective), conventional oncologists are basically shooting in the dark and hoping that they have designed the best protocol.

The patient also needs to keep in mind that if confronted by a physician or medical professional who insists that alternative therapies are not evidence-based medicine, he or she should counter either mentally or verbally that only 20% to 30% of what doctors do on a daily basis has been subjected to evidence-based medicine.

Any time a patient is on more than two prescription drugs daily, there is no evidence-based study proving anything. This statement was made by Stephen Chernisky, former professor of nutritional sciences at the University of California, Los Angeles (UCLA). He further states: "Big Pharma rarely runs studies on patients taking more than two drugs at a time, and drug interactions for poly-pharmacy are virtually unknown and untested."

After assimilating these and other related facts in the preceding chapter, the wise cancer patient now has no other rational option than to seriously consider seeking a consultation with a specialist in integrative oncology.

CHAPTER 4

CANCER

An Overview and How Traditional Treatments Are Failing to Treat It

Before we delve into the many possible causes of cancer, it's important to understand what exactly cancer is, how it develops, and how it spreads through your body.

A cancer cell is one in which the nuclear DNA is altered or damaged by a multitude of factors (to be described later). This damage leads to a faulty code that continues to replicate itself, and thus produces a continuous array of similar altered cells that grow geometrically in an out-of-control fashion.

These cells are not responsive to regulations by the hormonal, neural, or immune systems and are basically renegade cells. These renegades spread out of control and begin to invade not only the organs they are derived from, but also neighboring tissue. This growth may be slow and indolent, with doubling times greater than one year, or rapid, with doubling times measured in weeks or even days.

In general, cancers derived from blood-forming organs, such as lymphomas, myelomas, and leukemias, have the fastest doubling times. The growing mass of cancer cells show no consideration for its neighbors, including the supporting tissues, muscle tissues, nerves, blood vessels, and bony structures.

Eventually these renegade cells reach the streets and highways of the body: the lymphatic channels, the veins, the arteries, and the perineural spaces (nerves and nervous tissue). After access to these circulating channels, the cancer cells have the ability to flourish—like an acorn that after being carried in a stream comes to rest on a bank and grows into an oak tree— spreading to the major organs of the body, such as the brain, lungs, liver, and bones.

This migration of the cancer is called metastases. When new lesions arise in these final destination sites, the disease is termed Stage IV. There is no higher stage than a Stage IV cancer, so it is often used in conjunction with the terms "advanced cancer" or "incurable cancer."

Of cancers that have reached Stage IV, most oncology trainees are told, "You can't chase cancer with a scalpel or a radiation beam." For the great majority of cases, this pronouncement is correct. Once cancer is circulating through the system, the entire body is at risk and all treatment modalities must be systemic in nature.

In the case of Stage IV cancers, systemic therapy combining chemotherapy, immunotherapy, targeted therapies, and even nutritional therapies is the patient's last resort for any chance, however small, at a curative outcome.

If there is anything on which conventional and integrative oncologists, along with research scientists, agree unequivocally, it's that the causes of the many types of cancer afflicting humankind are complex and involve multiple factors, most within our control but some outside of it. However, it seems as though most traditional oncologists are uninterested in looking for triggers to determine what caused your cancer. This is the wrong way to go about diagnosis and treatment.

Often it is the synergy of many factors, both haphazardly and in concert, that allow a cancer to develop and gain a foothold in the human body. Some scientists analogize the takeover of a cancer in an individual to the takeover of an orderly society by rebellious elements that recruit more and more revolutionarily minded individuals. The healthy human body, like an orderly society, at all times has cancer cells searching for ways to destroy and kill by increasing their population.

At any given time thousands of cancer cells, out of the trillions of cells in the body, are searching for ways to exact harm by growing and spreading, and by destroying and weakening healthy cells, thereby creating a number of symptoms in the human host, including bouts of pain, weakness, lack of energy, nausea, vomiting, diarrhea, bleeding, and weight loss. A weakened immune system also heightens susceptibility to bacterial, fungal, viral, and parasitic infections.

Our major defense against these rebellious cells is an intact immune system. The immune system contains the B cells, of bone marrow origin, and the T cells (the so-called helper and suppressor cells), of thymus origin. Along with these frontline troops are the natural killer cells, which originate in the bone marrow and are capable of destroying the invading cancer cells upon contact.

The importance of this magnificent defense system was brought into clearer focus with the AIDS epidemic, which began in the 1970s but was not scientifically defined until the early 1980s in research laboratories in France and the United States. This deadly retrovirus was found to be capable of destroying and inactivating the B cell population of the human body.

The attack on this vital component of the immune system opened the gates to not only a number of serious viral, fungal, bacterial, and parasitic infections, but also a wide variety of cancers heretofore rarely seen in young adults. These included Kaposi's sarcoma, primary lymphomas of the brain, head and neck cancers, cervical and anal cancers, liver cancers, and Hodgkin's disease. From these cases it became abundantly clear that a dysfunctional immune system was a key factor in causation of cancer.

GENES PLAY A LIMITED ROLE

In the past forty years a large portion of the more than $100 billion spent on cancer research has gone to prove the importance of genetic factors involved in cancer causation. Despite the hundreds of studies that have been conducted, little clinically useful information has been gained and it has become clear that inherited factors play a major role in no more than 3% to 5% of all cancers.

Perhaps the most clinically useful genetic test yet developed for cancer prevention is the test for the BRCA1 and BRCA2 mutations, which can alert females that they and possibly their female family members are at risk for developing breast and ovarian cancers.

FAILURE OF CONVENTIONAL CANCER THEORY

The fact that the age-adjusted mortality rate for most adult cancers has not significantly improved in the last 70 years suggests that the basic approach to destroying tumors using radical surgeries, devastating radiation treatments, and full-dose multiple drug chemotherapy has been a dismal failure.

Conventional treatment, based on the theory that removing a tumor surgically or with radiation therapy is the best method for "keeping the tumor in check" and preventing cancer recurrence, completely disregards the important physiologic characteristics of the cancer itself, which are the following four things:

Cancer cells metabolize anaerobically, meaning they do so without oxygen.

Cancer growth is inhibited by an alkaline pH level.

Cancer growth is inhibited by hyperoxygenation.

Cancer cells have the ability to grow utilizing only simple sugars.

In essence, when the doctors who do conventional treatments ignore these factors by overlooking the importance of diet, supplements, alkalinization, and bio-oxidative therapies—they are failing to treat the whole patient.

Most patients grasp the fact that the "gold standard" for finding cancer anywhere in the body is the PET scan (positron emission tomography), which uses a radio-tagged sugar molecule to "light up" cancer wherever it is hiding in the body. A sugar molecule is used because cancer loves simple sugars— each cancer cell is endowed with more insulin receptors than normal cells. It seems unbelievable, then, that oncologists don't ask patients to go on a low-sugar diet. Why conventional allopathic oncologists refuse to tell patients this obvious fact defies logic and constitutes still another reason to seek an integrative practitioner for treatment.

TYPES OF CANCER

While most cancers fall into the "big four" of lung, prostate, breast, and colorectal cancers, there are actually 150 different histologic and pathologic varieties of cancers. They fall into three major varieties or categories:

(1) Carcinomas. These derive embryologically from the early ectodermal tissues and consist of cells that either cover or line various body surfaces or comprise major organs. This group includes all head and neck cancers, esophageal cancers, gastric cancers, small bowel cancers and colorectal cancers, as well as anal cancers. It also includes cells lining the trachea, bronchial tubes, and the lung itself. Carcinomas include cancers arising in all major organs, such as the thyroid gland, adrenal glands, liver, kidneys, ureters, bladder, and prostate, as well as the testes and ovaries.

(2) Sarcomas. Of mesodermal origin, sarcomas are composed of connective and supportive tissues such as bone, fibrous tissue, muscle tissue, blood vessel tissues, joint tissues, cartilage, and nerve tissues, as well as mixtures of all of the above. Most breast cancers are carcinomas, and the breast tissue itself contains small ductules that are the source of most breast cancers; rarely, though, a sarcoma will develop in the breast-supportive tissues. These constitute less than 2% of all breast cancers.

(3) Blood, or hemopoietic, cancers. These arise in lymph tissue, the spleen, the thymus gland, the bone marrow tissues, in various white blood cell components, and in red blood cell precursors. Hemopoietic cancers have specific names based on their points of origin: myelomas, from bone marrow; thymomas, from thymus tissue; lymphomas, both Hodgkin's type and non-Hodgkin's type, arising from the lymph nodes and spleen; and acute and chronic forms of leukemias, arising from white-blood-cell and red-blood-cell stem cells.

The staging of a cancer to assess its progression may be done by the oncologist, surgeon, or radiation therapist based on the size of the primary tumor, the degree of spread to regional nodes, the spread to more distant lymph node sites, and the spread to major organs including the brain, lungs, liver, and bone structures.

The grading of a tumor is usually done by the pathologist at the time of the initial biopsy. A grade 1 cancer appears less malignant with fewer mitoses under the microscope than a grade 4 cancer, in which the cells have more mitoses and a more undifferentiated appearance.

The pathologist also looks at the biopsy for invasion of the cancer through the capsule of the involved organ or into lymphatic, venous channels, and perineural spaces. The pathologist must comment on the closeness of the biopsy specimen to the three-dimensional margins of the cancer because the proximity of a cancer to the margin of resection will determine for the surgeon if a repeat biopsy is required. It is also predictive of the likelihood of obtaining a cure from surgery alone.

COLLATERAL DAMAGE TO YOUR BODY AND HOW TO AVOID IT

When conventional oncologists talk about treating cancer, they usually mean a treatment that destroys the building blocks of the so-called "genetic blueprint," or to be more specific, the stem cells containing the DNA molecule itself.

The problem with this approach is that rather than taking aim specifically at dividing cancer cells, these treatments cause collateral damage to *any* cell in the body that is replicating itself. It is estimated that every twenty-four hours more than 300 billion cells replicate themselves in the human body, so we are talking about a lot of potential collateral injury.

These dividing cells are mostly surface cells that cover and line body surfaces such as the skin, hair follicles, and the entire lining of the respiratory tract from the nasal mucosa to the cells lining the most distal alveolar air sacs. These are also the cells that line the entire surface of the alimentary tract from the oral mucosa to the anal surface. They include all of the cells derived from the blood or hematopoietic system, including the red blood cells, platelets, B and T cells, and the natural killer cells, as well as all the many individual components of the white blood cell system.

During the past twenty years, treatments that are directly targeted at lymphocyte subclasses (including CD-20 and CD-54) have been developed and used successfully, along with specific receptors on malignant cells referred to as epithelial growth factor receptors, or EGFR. Enzyme inhibitors called tyrosine kinase inhibitors and proteostome inhibitors have also become available as treatments.

Specific targeted therapies involve treatments with vascular endothelial growth factors (VEGF) to inhibit the growing cancer from creating its own blood supply, which it does to allow the invading cancer cells to survive.

In other words, a growing cancer needs oxygen and nutrition. It also requires a waste disposal system to carry away the waste products of cellular destruction, as well as the carbon dioxide, which is the end product of cellular respiration. The VEGF therapy interrupts that flow, and the cancer cell starves.

*

Given the advances that have occurred in cancer treatments, it is difficult to understand why cancer researchers and clinical oncologists have been unable to predict or identify a single factor, and by extrapolation a single treatment or group of treatments, that is 100% effective for any individual cancer.

Without a holistic approach or attention to the body's inherent physiology and biochemistry, appropriate treatment protocols used by conventional oncology are unlikely to produce lasting remissions, or more importantly, cures.

CHAPTER FIVE

WHAT DO CHEMO DRUGS CONTRIBUTE?

Prior to the late 1940s, the term "chemotherapy" was unknown, which shouldn't be surprising since even as late as the early 1960s, there were no medical oncology courses in most medical schools. The first board certification for medical oncology was not offered until 1972, so it is a relatively new specialized field of medicine.

The intended purpose of chemotherapeutic agents in the treatment of cancer is to prevent cancer cells from multiplying, invading, and metastasizing, and from ultimately killing the patient. Most chemotherapeutic agents currently in use appear to exert their primary effect on cell multiplication and tumor growth.

The problem is that most chemotherapeutic agents have considerable toxic effect on healthy cells, too, as they target *all* cells that multiply, whether cancer cells or healthy cells. Cell multiplication is a characteristic of more than 300 billion cells in our body per day, which includes cancer cells but also includes normal cells.

Cells with rapid rates of turnover are those most aggressively targeted by chemotherapeutic agents; a prime example are the short-lived bone marrow cells, which contain precursors of red cells, white cells, platelets, macrophages, and plasma cells. The cells lining the gastrointestinal tract have a rapid rate of turnover as well, due to wear and tear from digestive processes, acid and enzyme exposure, and exposure to bacterial growth in the lower portions of the colon. Also subject to high turnover rates—and thus at risk from chemotherapeutic agents—are the cells lining the respiratory tract, from the sinuses through the mucous membranes lining the mouth, nose, posterior pharynx, larynx, tracheobronchial tree, and ultimately the alveolar air sacs; all are under considerable wear and tear from repetitive respiratory rates averaging between 16 and 24 breaths per minute.

With few exceptions, the reasons that chemotherapeutic agents are more effective against cancer cells than normal cells are not well understood. Most chemotherapy agents interfere with either the synthesis of DNA, RNA, or proteins, or with parts of the division cycle and division spindle.

Chemotherapy today may involve single-agent therapy, in which the single best drug (according to clinical studies) is used, or combination therapy, in which two or more drugs are used in order to prevent resistance by zeroing in on the cancer cells, both when they are in their dividing phase and in their resting phase.

A number of biologic agents have been developed within the past three decades to stimulate immune function. This group of agents is called biologic response modifiers (BRMs). Some major BRMs used in cancer treatment include interferons, interleukins, colony stimulating factors, and a few others that are attached to radioactive compounds. These are agents used in addition to or in conjunction with chemotherapy.

In the late 1940s military pathologists performing autopsies on soldiers who were exposed to nitrogen mustard gasses and compounds found them to have extreme damage to vital bone marrow elements. The bone marrow cellular structure was often completely shorn of any red cell or white cell precursors. From this finding, it was extrapolated that nitrogen mustard compounds and analogs of these compounds could possibly be used to attack bone marrow malignancies such as leukemias and lymphomas.

Thus was introduced the first semi-successful group of drugs for the treatment of cancer, known as alkylating agents. This group of drugs multiplied over the next six decades and now includes the following drug agents: chlorambucil, cyclophosphamide, ifosfamide, mustargen and melphalan. Additional drugs in this category include busulfan, carmustine, lomustine and dacarbazine.

Platinum-containing drugs, which were discovered and brought into therapeutic usage in the 1980s, are part of this alkylating agents group as well, and include cisplatin, carboplatin, and oxaliplatin.

These alkylating agents are still widely used today and are effective for treatment of the following diseases:

1. Hodgkin's disease
2. Non-Hodgkin's lymphoma
3. Breast cancer
4. Small-cell lung cancer
5. Primary brain cancers
6. Various sarcomas
7. Chronic leukemias
8. Ovarian cancers
9. Esophageal and gastric cancers
10. Myelomas
11. Head and neck cancers

In the late 1940s and early 1950s, cancer research concentrated on the development of anti-metabolite drugs. These agents were designed to interfere with the building blocks of the DNA and RNA molecules. The earliest of these drugs were methotrexate, 6-mercaptopurine, thioguanine, cytarabine, flu-orouracil, and Fludara.

This family of drugs still finds usage today for treatment of the following:

1. Head and neck cancers
2. Esophageal cancer
3. Pancreatic cancer
4. Gastric cancer
5. Breast cancer
6. Colorectal cancer
7. Anal cancer
8. Acute leukemias
9. Chronic leukemias

In the 1960s, after testing procedures were accomplished, discoveries were made revealing that natural products from herbal derivatives showed very favorable efficacy. Among these was the vinca group of drugs, which were termed "mitotic inhibitors" and included vinblastine, vincristine, and VP-16. These drugs work by inhibiting the division of cancer cells.

After the mitotic inhibitors, a number of antibiotic-related chemotherapy agents came into usage in the early 1970s. These drugs include bleomycin, daunomycin, dactinomycin, doxorubicin, idarubicin, mithramycin, mitomycin, and mitoxantrone.

This group of drugs is widely used, even today in modern medical oncology, for:

1. Primary brain tumors
2. Hodgkin's disease
3. Non-Hodgkin's lymphoma
4. Breast cancer
5. Bladder cancer
6. Various sarcomas
7. Melanomas
8. Testicular cancers
9. Ovarian cancers
10. Pancreatic cancer
11. Anal cancers

In the early 1970s, yet another class of drugs, known as the nitrosoureas, which acted like alkylating agents, were developed. The main agents in this group included BCNU and CCNU. These agents proved useful then and are still in use today for treatment of the following:

1. Primary brain tumors
2. Hodgkin's disease
3. Lymphomas
4. Melanomas
5. Sarcomas

From the 1980s through the year 2000, the two most impor-tant classes of chemotherapy agents to emerge in standard on-cology treatment protocols were the platinum compounds (as mentioned earlier in this chapter, cisplatin, carboplatin, and oxaliplatin) and the taxane compounds.

The taxane group, derived from the bark of the yew tree, included Taxol, Taxotere, and Abraxane. The combination of these two new classes is now the leading, first-line protocol for treating the following:

1. Non-small-cell lung carcinoma
2. Ovarian carcinoma
3. Head and neck tumors
4. Hormone-independent prostate cancer
5. Testicular cancers
6. Esophageal and gastric cancers

Other less-significant agents, some dating back to the early 1970s, were introduced but have seen less usage in modern medical oncology. A number of hormonal agents and hormone antagonists have been useful, dating way back to the 1950s and 1960s, which include:

1. Various androgens
2. Corticosteroids

3. Estrogens

4. Progestational agents

5. Estrogen antagonists

6. Androgen antagonists

7. Luteinizing hormone/releasing-hormone antagonists (LHRH)

8. Aromatase inhibitors

To add to this mixture, there are several miscellaneous agents that are also available for treating specific types of cancers:

- The drug asparaginase is a specific enzyme used only in childhood lymphocytic leukemia.
- The drug hydroxyurea is useful in chronic myelogenous leukemias and in brain cancers.
- A jet-fuel derivative called procarbazine is still used today in Hodgkin's disease and in certain brain tumors.
- A specific adrenocortical suppressive agent called mitotane is useful in the rare adrenocortical cancers.
- A drug called aminoglutethimide is a steroid synthesis inhibitor.
- And lastly, the drug altretamine is useful as a tertiary (a third or fourth line chemotherapy option) agent in ovarian cancer.

During the first decade of the twenty-first century, targeted therapies specific to treatment of certain molecular components of the cancer cells themselves—specifically epithelial growth factor receptors (EGFR), vascular endothelial growth factors (VEGF), and tyrosine kinase inhibitors (TKIs)—were developed. Drugs in these categories are the latest and most specific available for use in major cancers, and are as close as we have ever come in medical oncology to using specific drugs for specific cancer cell characteristics. These drugs include:

1. Iressa
2. Tarceva
3. Erbitux
4. Avastin
5. Nexavar
6. Sutent
7. The mTOR family of drugs

The use of these agents has been the most useful in:

1. Primary brain tumors
2. Head and neck cancers
3. Non-small-cell lung cancers
4. Breast cancers
5. Ovarian cancers
6. Renal cell cancers
7. Primary liver cancers
8. Neuroendocrine tumors
9. Pancreatic cancers

Despite all the publicized successes, there is still a dark side to the evolution of these "super drugs." While many have been helpful and many have been hyped as panaceas, the truth is that often, the actual benefit from using them is an increased survival duration of only three to six months.

The drug adriamycin, for example, which can cause significant cardiac function impairments, may be useless in estrogen-positive breast cancer patients despite the fact that it has been used extensively over the past 30 years as the frontline adjuvant therapy for Stage II breast cancers and for metastatic breast cancer disease.

Another drug, Iressa, touted as an orally targeted treatment for non-small-cell lung cancer, and a drug that, for four years, was on the market at a price of more than $20,000 per year to uninsured patients, has been found in follow-up studies to be no better than a placebo in the treatment of non-small-cell lung cancer.

To reiterate, conventional oncologists routinely administer powerful toxic chemotherapy drugs to cancer patients based on statistical probabilities that these drugs will have a positive effect on shrinking the cancer and moving the patient into a complete, partial, or stable disease state. If they are wrong, as often happens, the patient is essentially taking a poison without any beneficial effects. What this means is that when ineffective chemotherapy is given, the patient must endure all of the toxicities without receiving any benefits whatsoever.

Additionally, the devastating side effects of multi-drug chemotherapy on the brain, heart, liver, kidneys, and nervous system raise quality of life issues for those few patients who survive five years of chemotherapy for Stage IV disease. Is it worth the expense and the toxic side effects you will experience from reliance on these drugs for the chance that you will be one of only 2 out of 100 patients alive after five years? If there was no other alternative course of treatment, the answer to that question might reasonably be yes. But as you will see in Part Two of this book, alternatives do exist in the field of integrative medicine—alternatives that can preserve quality of life while extending the length of that life.

CHAPTER SIX

NUMBERS DETAIL
A HISTORY OF FAILURE

Probably the most damning evidence demonstrating the limitations and deficiencies of conventional cancer treatment can be found in two categories of statistics: (1) the annual rate of newly diagnosed cancer cases, and (2) the survival rates of patients battling the "big four" of lung, prostate, breast, and colorectal cancers.

The many costs of cancer, especially the pain and suffering that this disease causes, can't be adequately expressed in mere statistics and numbers. But the litany of lives lost and the amount of public and private monies spent fighting this health scourge do provide a convenient yardstick by which to measure whether we've made progress with traditional treatments.

Seventy years ago, when I was a child, only one in thirty patients died of cancer; today this number is two in three. The World Health Organization reports that as of 2010, cancer remained the leading cause of death worldwide.

The War on Cancer in the US, which began during the Nixon administration in the early 1970s, has been an embarrassingly dismal failure at a cost to taxpayers of over $100 billion, mostly spent on projects to research variations on the "slash-and-burn" approach to treatment. During the past forty years, the number of new cancers has steadily increased and conventional treatments have failed to adequately improve the rate of overall survivability.

Very little progress has been made in conventional oncology in treating the big four cancers. There has been almost no significant breakthrough in liver cancers, pancreatic cancers, renal cell cancers, or melanomas. Most disturbing is the impact on the most innocent and vulnerable among us—childhood cancers have increased by 30% since the government-funded War on Cancer was declared.

Cancer cases diagnosed in the United States today approach 1.5 million per year, with more than 560,000 deaths annually. Since the War on Cancer was declared:

- malignant skin cancer (melanoma) increased by more than 80%
- non-Hodgkin's lymphoma cases escalated by 50%
- lung cancers went up by 35%, making this the deadliest form of cancer today
- there has been a more than 600% increase in prostate

cancer diagnoses; today, one in six men will develop
prostate cancer

American Cancer Society statistics reveal that the big four
cancer survival rate in the past twenty years increased by only
2%, whereas the survival rate for liver, lung, pancreas, and
kidney cancers has not improved significantly for the past four
decades. This is truly a grim reality.

There is not yet a "magic bullet" that treats all cancers, nor
is there any cancer that responds 100% to any single drug or
group of drugs. The onslaught of "slash-and-burn" tactics used
in combating cancer leaves the body's intrinsic defense mech-
anisms—immune function, white blood cells, natural killer
cells, B and T cells—all totally depleted.

One cannot help but conclude that the steady increase in
cancer deaths from 1971 to the present mutes any claim of vic-
tory in the War on Cancer. If anything, we must conclude that
conventional "slash-and-burn" cancer treatments—coupled
with a lack of attention to all factors involved in disease prevention—have produced little progress in alleviating the pain and
suffering of a cruel disease that continues its devastating ero-
sion of human health and longevity.

Based on the poor results of current conventional cancer
treatments, the successful oncologist of the future should
widen his or her horizons and consider a new path for treatment. In Part Two, I will detail these already available, less-
toxic alternatives that are more effective in killing the cancer
without killing the patient in the process. The successful oncologist of the future must address the whole person, their
emotional profile, their nutritional needs, their supplemental

needs, the detoxification of their underlying heavy-metal and chemical toxins, the integrity of their immune system, their dental health, and most of all, protect their entire anatomical, physiological, and biochemical systems from undue toxicity and from excessive amounts of radiation, surgery, and massive doses of chemotherapy.

CHAPTER SEVEN

FIVE MYTHS ABOUT CONVENTIONAL CANCER TREATMENTS

→ **MYTH #1:** You need to show adverse effects such as nausea, vomiting, diarrhea, skin rashes, or bone marrow suppression in order to know that chemotherapy is really working.

→ **FACTS:** The extent to which you poison your body isn't a standard by which to judge whether cancer treatment will be effective or not. Low-dose fractionated chemotherapy, or insulin potentiated therapy, rarely create toxic side effects so commonly seen with high-dose chemo, yet these approaches are still effective in fighting the advance of cancer, as I will describe in Part Two of this book.

➜ **MYTH #2:** You must never deviate from any chemotherapy protocol once started, if you are to achieve optimal results.

➜ **FACTS:** The taxanes, the anthracyclines, and several platinum drugs that are currently on the market were originally given to patients at three-week intervals. After years of use and study of their effects on patients, lower weekly doses have become the prescribing rule. (More about that later.)

➜ **MYTH #3:** A cancer patient must always use high-dose chemotherapy in order to obtain optimal results.

➜ **FACTS:** The original Xeloda dosage recommendations were so high that this oral chemotherapy agent, given every 14 out of 21 days in a cyclic fashion, caused severe stomatitis and hand-foot syndrome, resulting in severe pain and swelling of the palms of the hands and soles of the feet. Through trial and error, a lower dose coupled with week-on/week-off distribution method became the preferred treatment option.

➜ **MYTH #4:** The platinum-containing chemotherapy drugs—cisplatin, carboplatin, and oxaliplatin—don't cause long-term disabilities to users.

➜ **FACTS:** Cancer patients who undergo routine hair analysis for toxic metals consistently show that prior treatment with platinum-containing chemotherapy agents produces high levels of toxicity in the body, accompanied by physical impairments. These impairments include hearing loss, kidney damage, and sensory nerve damage.

➔ **MYTH #5:** It doesn't matter what cancer patients eat, so they shouldn't be discouraged from consuming chocolates and other "comfort foods."

➔ **FACTS:** In the 1930s, Otto Warburg, MD, discovered that cancer cells thrive on simple sugars, a revelation which earned him a Nobel Prize in Medicine. Since then his discovery about the relationship between cancer growth and sugar has been verified in a variety of ways.

For instance, consider what happens with the PET scan, which is the "gold standard" for finding cancer anywhere in the human body. It's based upon a radio-tagged sugar molecule "lighting up" cancer wherever it may be found in the body. Cancer cells have many more insulin receptors than normal cells, which accounts for their ability to grab onto the radio-tagged sugar molecules. This nuclear medicine procedure, in itself, demonstrates that sugar is essential for malignant cell survival, which means that a low-sugar diet is essential to long-term recovery

➔ **MYTH #6:** Rationed care will lower costs and benefit cancer patients. Though this one hasn't evolved into a widespread myth yet, it deserves to be addressed before it does, because it's highly unlikely that rationed care will improve overall survival rates for cancer patients.

➔ **FACTS:** *Untermenschen* is a German word meaning "less than human," which was used by Adolf Hitler's Third Reich in the 1930s to create a category of human beings who were considered to be no longer useful, productive, tax-paying citizens.

This group included the chronically ill, the insane, the elderly, and the physically and mentally disabled.

Hitler used rationed care and death panels to discard these individuals, either by restricting their medical care or by introducing various forms of euthanasia, in order to rid Germany of this unwanted tax burden so it could climb out of the worldwide Depression of the 1930s.

While this is maybe the most extreme example ever of rationing and death panels, the concept of rationed care and cost-containment panels has begun to resurface in subtle ways under the Patient Protections and Affordable Care Act.

Some of the health-care policy changes affecting cancer prevention and treatment since 2010 have included:

1. Restrictions of expensive targeted cancer drugs for advanced cancers, based largely on cost considerations.
2. Raising the age of approved PAP smear testing in women from 18 years of age to 21 years of age.
3. Restricted payments for screening mammograms for women over the age of 75.
4. Non-treatment of early prostate cancer in men over the age of 50 with increased prostate-specific antigen (PSA) levels, relying instead on "watchful waiting."
5. Allowing coverage of only generic drugs for Medicaid and Medicare patients.

Many of these restrictions, and more, are already the rule in Canada, England, and other countries that practice forms of socialized medicine. But have these policies really contained costs, except at the expense of quality care?

One philosophy that is surfacing early in the Patient

Protection and Affordable Care Act is that the use of expensive drugs for cancer or other diseases may not be affordable by any health-care system where a definitive cure is non-obtainable.

This "by the numbers" approach takes into account all of the expenses incurred in treating a patient with advanced disease that isn't curable by primary surgery or radiation therapy alone. These costs include the total expenses and duration of treatment with chemotherapy as well as the expected expenses associated with the adverse toxicities related to the initial therapies. It also includes all of the radiological and laboratory costs for monitoring these patients, along with the costs of medical visits and infusion center visits.

This is at best a numbers game. Because every patient is unique and will respond differently to various choices of chemotherapy drugs and even to palliative radiation therapy treatments, it's impossible to visualize any complex calculus formula that could ever take all of these variables into consideration.

Despite this, the federal government, through the Department of Health & Human Services, has developed the Incremental Cost-Effectiveness Ratio (ICER), which purportedly gives the "cost per quality-adjusted life year" gained. Providing the decision-making panels with numbers is the ultimate goal of the HHS so that a judgment can be made on either allowing or withholding certain therapies.

For example: A renal failure patient on dialysis is estimated by the ICER formula to cost, on average, $129,000 per year.

The Swiss health-care system has concluded that the anti-angiogenesis drug Avastin costs $43,000 for only 0.35 Quality-Adjusted Life Years (QALY). This is equal to an ICER of about $125,000 of QALY per year.

The question is, does any individual deserve to have his or

her life span determined (or limited) by a formula that may or may not be accurate?

Reducing individuals to a set of statistics has become accepted practice. So much so that a recent television commercial for UnitedHealthcare shows a jogger with various numbers scrolling up and down her body, detailing her vital signs, age, cholesterol level, renal function, liver function, blood counts, and other numerical parameters. At the end of the commercial a voice states, "UnitedHealthcare...medicine by the numbers."

Does any thoughtful physician believe we can pigeonhole patients into certain categories by numbers alone? Can anyone truly make a persuasive case that rationed care will help to cure cancer?

THE ECONOMIC AND HUMAN TOLL OF CANCER WORLDWIDE

Without a doubt, the growing economic toll of the worldwide cancer epidemic continues unabated. This financial burden will increasingly affect developing countries and place excessive demands on their health-care systems. The economies of these countries will not be able to bear these financial burdens and rationing will be the result, as we're already seeing in the United States.

Cancer is the leading cause of death worldwide, surpassing malaria, tuberculosis, and HIV combined. The worldwide price tag is thought to be about $1 trillion annually. It is estimated by the American Cancer Society that the number of new cases of cancer will double by the year 2030, just twenty years from now.

According to a 2008 World Health Organization (WHO) study of 188 countries and 17 different forms of cancer:

- global economy losses from cancer, excluding direct treatment costs, totaled nearly $900 billion per year
- the US had the highest economic burden in absolute dollars
- the US lost 1.7% of its gross domestic product (GDP), whereas most developing countries lost greater than 2% to 3% of their GDP, because of cancer disabilities
- the cancers with the greatest economic impact were lung, colorectal, and breast cancers
- cancer caused more economic damage than any of the world's fifteen other leading causes of death: 20% higher than heart disease, the next leading cause of death

Taken together, these statistics make a compelling case that we must begin to reduce the costs to our health-care system of conventional cancer treatment policies that we no longer can afford. Real cost containment of treatment policies means prescribing fewer chemo drugs and less radiation, and implementing more cancer prevention education programs. Integrative oncology supports and offers society this approach. Conventional oncology does not.

2

YOUR

INTEGRATIVE

CANCER

TREATMENT

OPTION

CHAPTER EIGHT

WHAT IS INTEGRATIVE ONCOLOGY?

Common terms for the type of oncology that I practice include: alternative oncology, complementary oncology, and integrative oncology.

Of these, I prefer the name integrative oncology, as I feel that this most accurately describes my practice, which is to combine the best of both worlds—namely, conventional protocol-based chemotherapy and complementary therapy, which augments chemotherapy with the safe, nontoxic alternative therapies.

My message to you about this form of disease treatment is simple, poignant, and direct: successful and life-saving cancer therapy can be accomplished using integrative cancer medicine!

My promise to you is that the discouraging and dismal results seen from the use of chemotherapy for Stage IV cancers
can be improved upon more than twentyfold using the information contained in the following pages.

When patients ask about a cure for their cancer, as an integrative oncologist I tell them that a cure, medically speaking, is
an equation: complete remission (the absence of any measurable cancer by all technologies) plus time (usually five years or
more) equals cure.

The caveat here is that there are a number of cancers that lie
dormant for many years, even five to twenty years after being
in complete remission. These cancers typically include breast
cancer, melanomas, thyroid cancer, and renal cell cancer, to
name just the most common.

Conventional oncology has always been searching for the
cure-all that will knock out all of these cancers. However, because of the multiple causative factors involved in initiating a
cancer, it is unlikely that conventional medicine will ever find
this "pot of gold" at the end of the rainbow.

Integrative oncology looks into the self-healing properties
of the body, as well as the molecular biology of the cancer cell
itself, incorporating the importance of sugar-free diets, alkalin-
izing diets, bio-oxidative therapies, specific vitamin therapies,
herbal therapies, and amino acid supplements.

Use of these modalities with low-dose fractionated chemotherapy and insulin potentiated therapies, in combination with
immune-stimulating and supportive therapies, will, in the long
run, contribute to a higher success rate with fewer side effects
and a less toxic burden on biological systems.

As I discussed earlier in this book, rarely do oncologists talk
about looking for the triggers to determine what caused the

cancer in the first place. Whether it is chemical exposures on the job, or the quality of diet consumed by the patient, these are the sorts of considerations that conventional oncologists seem unconcerned about, so preoccupied are they by their "slash and burn" treatment.

In stark contrast to the earlier discussion of what a conventional oncologist will do (or more likely not do) to determine the cause of your cancer, an integrative oncologist has a full arsenal of testing to do. Allergy testing, hair analysis, and other non-invasive tests can help to identify possible triggers for the cancer. An integrative oncologist wants to know all of this information to prevent the cancer from recurring once it goes into remission or is cured.

When a hair analysis finds high levels of mercury, tin, silver, and nickel, that usually refers to dental amalgams, so you advise the patient to have these metals removed once the cancer is dealt with, replacing the metals with nontoxic dental fillings. If a patient is tested and found to have high levels of heavy metals and other toxins, then he or she should undergo detoxification using any number of detoxification strategies after basic cancer treatment is underway. If mercury alone is elevated, that usually means a dietary source such as fish is the culprit.

Learning the cause of the cancer empowers patients. Receiving an answer to the "why me?" question helps them psychologically, especially if they have no genetic predisposition and family history for the disease. Additionally, identifying the cancer triggers can help to prevent a recurrence of the cancer that might otherwise result from re-exposure to the original toxins.

As you can see, in many ways integrative oncology ends up

being defined as treatments and therapies not provided by conventional oncology's slash-and-burn methods.

WHY IS INTEGRATIVE ONCOLOGY OPPOSED?

The reasons that there are precious few integrative oncologists in practice today in the United States are varied, but can be distilled into a few major ones.

Political and economic forces within the US stifle news favorable to alternative therapies because Big Pharma, the US Food and Drug Administration (FDA), the National Institutes of Health (NIH), and the National Cancer Institute (NCI) resist changes in our malfunctioning health-care system due to the enormous amounts of monies that are made by keeping the system exactly the way it is.

Most physicians are deaf to the reality that the politics and economics of cancer medicine trump the science of cancer medicine. Most conventional oncologists are oblivious to the poor results from long-term chemotherapy treatment of up to five years or more, and to the multiple adverse reactions in the human body that these drugs produce, which damage the quality of life of the patient's remaining life span.

But the number-one reason that integrative oncologists are so few, without a doubt, is the restrictions placed on doctors by the individual state medical boards and, in turn, by their overseers, the Federation of State Medical Boards. This entity is directly guided by the Food and Drug Administration, which in turn takes orders and gets major funding from Big Pharma.

The Big Pharma corporations are solely dedicated to manufacturing, distributing, and propagandizing drugs. Any substance that diagnoses, prevents, mitigates, treats, or cures any disease or condition under US law is considered a "drug." And yet, for some incomprehensible reason, various vitamins and minerals that mitigate, treat, and cure vitamin-deficiency diseases are *not* considered drugs, but rather natural substances. This reasoning is impossible to comprehend intellectually, as we know that diseases such as scurvy, beriberi, rickets, pellagra, and pernicious anemia can be cured with vitamins and minerals in appropriate doses.

By propagandizing to doctors and to patients directly through radio, television, and Internet advertising, Big Pharma attempts to sway physician and public opinion and encourage patients to request specific drugs from their primary care physicians. I bet you didn't know that the United States is the only country in the world, aside from New Zealand, that allows drug advertising by pharmaceutical companies.

Big Pharma's propaganda campaign also includes an army of drug representatives who shower physicians with gifts, including pens, paperweights, cups, calendars, lunches, dinners, various unhealthy snack foods, ties, clocks, and even vacations in attractive resort destinations.

These pharmaceutical industry methods have prompted some alternative doctors to compare the relationship between Big Pharma and many mainstream doctors to that of a pimp and his prostitutes. The acceptance of this propaganda helps to solidify mainstream medicine's aversion, if not active resistance, to integrative approaches to treatment that involve less reliance on pharmaceutical drugs.

PUBLIC DEMANDS FOR EXPANDED HEALTH-CARE OPTIONS

Despite scorn and opposition from Big Pharma and conventional medicine, alternative approaches to health care have never been more in demand by the public. Integrative oncology owes much to the growing field of complementary treatments, which continue to blossom around the world.

A landmark study published in the renowned *New England Journal of Medicine* in 1993 brought sunshine to this movement by providing the following statistics, based on interviews with more than 1,500 US citizens: one-third stated that they visited at least one alternative practitioner during the previous year; one-third had seen their alternative practitioner more than fifteen times in one year. The survey also revealed that more than 70% of patients seeing an "unconventional professional" kept this a secret from their primary-care physician.

During the 1990s, alternative medicine was the second fastest growing area of medicine, behind home health-care services. Further proof of the quickly burgeoning acceptance of complementary medicine comes from a poll by *Self* magazine during the last decade, which showed that 84% of their readers had consulted an unconventional practitioner and that 36% of their readers had more confidence in the care of alternative doctors than in allopathic doctors.

In terms of integrative oncology, surveys by the American Cancer Society have reported that 10% of Americans with cancer used complementary therapies, either alone or with conventional chemotherapy. Other studies carried out at a large university cancer center have reported that as many as

50% of cancer patients have tried some form of alternative or integrative therapy during the past year.

Considering that there are annually 1.5 million patients diagnosed with some form of cancer, if one uses only the most conservative estimates, then at least 10% of cancer patients use some form of alternative therapy. This equates to 150,000 cancer patients per year who are using some form of alternative care as part of their overall treatment protocol.

In Europe, the trend is even more impressive. A German study involving a poll of several hundred cancer patients at a large clinic showed that at least 60% had used some type of alternative therapy during their treatment program.

Demand seems to be creating supply. More than 30% of medical schools now offer curricula containing alternative medicine electives.

How much of an impact has this growing acceptance of integrative and alternative care among cancer patients had on cancer survival statistics? We can't know the full extent of that contribution to cures and remissions because the American Cancer Institute and similar record-keeping institutions still don't include statistics from outside their strictly conventional oncology circles.

A HISTORY OF INTEGRATIVE ONCOLOGY

To understand the history of integrative medicine in general, and integrative oncology in specific, the reader needs to become familiar with the term "medical maverick." A maverick in any field, whether medicine or science or politics, for that matter, is one who acts independently and single-mindedly and refuses due to personal beliefs to conform to prevailing customs, rules, or regulations. This individual behaves and runs his or her life based on personal principles, ethics, and beliefs.

In medicine, mavericks practice not only the science of medicine, but also the "art of medicine." The history of science often includes an underlying pattern of faulty reasoning. Throughout modern history, mavericks are the ones who pioneered and corrected these errors and beliefs, and replaced them with advanced discoveries.

They were often initially ridiculed and condemned as quacks, charlatans, and snake-oil salesmen. But wise and far-sighted historians will simply label them as visionary mavericks.

SOME MAVERICK PIONEERS

Revolutionary ideas often evolve outside prevailing belief systems:

Christopher Columbus was ridiculed for his belief that the earth was round.

Isaac Newton was dismissed for his theory of gravitation.

Giordano Bruno was burned at the stake for claiming that the earth was not the center of the universe.

Galileo was imprisoned for claiming that the earth revolved around the sun.

Dr. Ignaz Philipp Semmelweis was belittled for his theory of antisepsis in the prevention of childbed fever.

Louis Pasteur was ostracized by doubting scientists for his theories on immunization relating to anthrax and rabies infections.

Galen, the real father of modern medicine, had to flee Rome from the wrath of frenzied mobs because of his anatomical theories, which later proved correct.

Dr. William Harvey was disgraced as a physician for believing that blood was pumped by the heart and moved throughout the entire body through arteries.

Wilhelm Roentgen, who discovered X-rays, was hailed as a quack.

Another prominent physician, **Edward Jenner,** who developed the smallpox vaccine, was criticized for experimenting on children and was said to be given to quackery.

MODERN-ERA INTEGRATIVE MEDICINE MAVERICKS

The story of the giants in the modern era of integrative medicine and oncology cannot be told without mentioning **Dr. Linus Pauling,** who died in 1994. He was truly a man of enormous achievements. To list all of his scientific achievements would in itself require a book. The field of orthomolecular medicine owes its existence to him.

The term "orthomolecular" was first coined by Dr. Pauling in 1968, in a *Science* magazine article. The standard definition of this term is "the practice of preventing and treating disease by providing the body with optimal amounts of substances which are natural to the body."

Dr. Pauling's renowned works cover many areas of biology, biochemistry, and physics. He won the Nobel Prize in Chemistry in 1959 for describing the nature of the chemical bond. He won a second Nobel Prize—a Nobel Peace Prize—in 1962 for his work in preventing atmospheric testing of nuclear weapons.

Like mavericks of the past in the field of medicine, Dr. Pauling was criticized for recommending megadoses of vitamins, especially vitamin C, in the treatment of viral illnesses and cancer. Dr. Pauling's interest in vitamin C led him to the concept that this antioxidant vitamin could be useful in the treatment of cancers as well as viral illnesses.

In his lectures, Dr. Pauling is quoted as saying that "vitamin C is involved in a great number of biochemical reactions in the human body." He went on to explain that two of its major interactions are in the potentiation of the immune system and in aiding in the synthesis of collagens, the support structure of connective tissues and the vascular system. He also clarified the fact that most animals, except for humans, monkeys, and guinea pigs, make their own vitamin C, and therefore do not require this essential vitamin from extrinsic sources.

Dr. Pauling criticized federal regulations for daily vitamin requirements by stating that "man's RDA of vitamin C should actually be 200 times the government's stated standard for RDA, or at least 12 grams per day."

Another pioneering giant of integrative medicine, **Dr. Robert Cathcart III,** put Dr. Pauling's theories about vitamin C to the test. Dr. Cathcart earned his medical degree at the University of California at San Francisco in 1954, completed residency training in orthopedic surgery, and became famous for his renowned Cathcart hip prosthesis. Branching out from orthopedic surgery in the 1970s, Dr. Cathcart began applying Dr. Linus Pauling's teachings to the treatment of viral illnesses, including influenza, hepatitis, and later to HIV. Later in the 1980s, Dr. Cathcart was able to show the successful application of high doses of vitamin C in advanced cancer patients.

Harry Hoxsey, born in 1901, was the first successful promoter of the widely used complementary, nontoxic therapy for cancer, which is still in use today in the US, called the Hoxsey Therapy. Although never able to complete formal medical training, Hoxsey was a self-taught healing practitioner. The herbal elixir promoted by Hoxsey in the early and mid 1900s was actually developed by Harry's great-grandfather, who, as a horse breeder, observed sick horses selectively chewing on certain herbs in the pasture, which were then collected by his great-grandfather and made into a potion. This formula was passed down to Harry's father, a veterinarian who used the Hoxsey Therapy in his practice.

When Harry came of age, he used this same potion and began treating friends and neighbors in the area who had fallen ill from cancer. His successes were significant, to the point where word spread of his herbal tonic. Because of the stigma that he was an "herbal quack" and the prejudice against any alternative form of medicine, it became impossible for him to matriculate into medical school. So Harry practiced under other physicians as a medical assistant and had the first successful clinic in the United States treating various adult cancers, in Dallas, Texas, in the late 1920s and 1930s. The constituents of Hoxsey's Therapy include, even today, a proprietary mixture of potassium iodine, red clover, burdock root, cascara, barberries, prickly ash, and licorice.

Although never purchased by any major pharmaceutical house because natural products cannot be patented, this mixture remains today as a significant symbol of the success of herbal therapy in the treatment of cancer. It is used in clinics today primarily in Mexico, Central and South America, Europe, and Asia.

Renee Caisse, RN, a French-Canadian, is another colorful character in the history of integrative oncology and herbal medicine. Nurse Caisse's struggle to find a cure for cancer dates back to her late twenties, when as a ward nurse she attended to an elderly female patient in an Ontario hospital who had evidence on her chest wall of a previous cancer. Nurse Caisse was told by the patient the story of how thirty years earlier she had advanced breast cancer and was given an herbal mixture by a French-Canadian Indian medicine man. The mixture contained at least four herbs: slippery elm, burdock root, sheep sorrel, and turkey rhubarb.

The patient, now thirty years in remission, so impressed Nurse Caisse that she made it her life's mission to collect these herbs and experiment with different recipes to reproduce their remarkable healing qualities. It is said that she cured her own mother's liver cancer with the herbal brew. Today commercial forms of Nurse Caisse's product (her name spelled backwards,

Essiac tea) such as E-Tea and FlorEssence tea are marketed by a number of companies. This product is still used as a supplement in many different forms of adult cancers in integrative practices.

Dr. Ernest T. Krebs is probably second only to Harry Hoxsey in prominence as a developer of important natural weapons in the integrative oncologist's "war on cancer." In the 1930s and 1940s, Dr. Krebs (later joined by his biochemist son, Ernest Krebs Jr.) discovered that vitamin B-17 (also called laetrile, amygdalin, or nitriloside) played a positive role at stopping the growth of cancer. Big Pharma and their enforcement arm, the FDA, have been successful in tainting and disparaging vitamin B-17 as a "quack remedy" and have also closed down most laetrile clinics in the US.

Nevada and Oklahoma are the only states in which laetrile remains legal. The unfortunate caveat to this is the law states that the substance must be manufactured in the State of Nevada only and Oklahoma doesn't recognize homeopathy, which is the only kind of medicine that generally uses laetrile. But because no compounding pharmacy (one which mixes its own drugs) in Nevada manufactures laetrile, laetrile patients must purchase their own supply outside of Nevada, and as such it is only rarely given intravenously in the state by alternative doctors working under the radar.

Interestingly enough, laetrile is the concentrated form of vitamin B-17 and is found in many foods commonly eaten, including almonds, berries, bean sprouts, apricot seeds, peach seeds, cherry seeds, and buckwheat. The apricot pit is the highest source of vitamin B-17 in the human diet. Populations of humans around the world who register high levels of vitamin

B-17 from their diet tend to demonstrate low incidence rates of cancer.

The biochemistry of the laetrile molecule consists of a glyco-benzaldehyde molecule with a cyanide molecule attachment. The cyanide can only be released by a specific enzyme possessed by cancer cells called beta-glucosidase. Thus, exposure of vitamin B-17 to cancer cells delivers a fatal punch to the cancer cells specifically and does not harm normal cells, which are protected by another enzyme called rhodanese.

Dr. John Richardson, who practiced medicine in the Bay Area of northern California and later moved to Reno, Nevada, along with his protégée **Dr. W. Douglas Brodie** (from the Bay Area and later Lake Tahoe and then Reno, Nevada), was an enthusiastic advocate for laetrile therapy during the sixties and seventies. Dr. Brodie was both an MD and a homeopathic medical doctor. Both of these physicians were harassed by the California Medical Society, and yet they continued treating patients with advanced cancers until each of them died while actively practicing.

One of the major arguments against vitamin B-17 was that it was "too toxic" because it contained a cyanide molecule. However, it seems that the cancer establishment forgot to mention that vitamin B-12, which is still in widespread use by allopathic physicians today, also contains a cyanide molecule and is essential to the prevention of pernicious anemia and combined systems disease. It is also water-soluble and virtually nontoxic, even if given in massive daily doses.

What is rarely mentioned by straight-line conventional oncologists and by members of the cancer establishment is that platinum-containing chemotherapy agents known by the names of cisplatin, carboplatin, and oxaliplatin leave behind residual toxicities much greater than any toxicity ever reported for vitamin B-17. These severe toxicities include ototoxicity (decreased hearing), nephrotoxicity (decreased renal function), and neurotoxicity (sensory damage to peripheral nerves). It should be noted that these toxicities may be either long-lasting or permanent.

According to Big Pharma and the cancer industry, death from chemotherapy is acceptable as long as standard protocol chemotherapy has been adhered to.

In Dr. Ralph W. Moss's book *The Cancer Industry*, he reports a deliberate cover-up by major cancer centers, including Sloan-Kettering Memorial Hospital in New York City, to hide the successful benefits of laetrile when this natural substance was experimented with in animal studies.

OTHER INFLUENTIAL FIGURES

In addition to the above giants in the field of integrative medicine and oncology, there is a long list of alternative medicine doctors who, although not all trained oncologists, have changed their practices to emphasize integrative oncology and have been successful in doing so. It's not in the scope of this book to write a detailed biography of all these heroes but rather to briefly mention their names and include their contact numbers in the appendix.

This list includes **Dr. Keith Block** of the Block Medical Center in Evanston, Illinois. Dr. Block's major philosophy is to flush toxins from the body and clean the liver, kidneys, lungs, lymph system, and skin. His clinic offers nutritional support and major organ support, as well as psychosocial support. He uses conventional chemotherapy to reduce the tumor burden while strengthening the body's intrinsic immune system.

Dr. W. John Diamond, a recently deceased pathologist by training, as well as a homeopathic practitioner, promoted homeopathic remedies combined with detoxification strategies. His protocols promoted nutritional supplementation, biological dentistry, and neural therapies.

Dr. Michael B. Schlachter trained as a psychiatrist at Columbia College of Physicians and Surgeons in New York, but later became excited by the prospect of using alternative treatments in the battle against cancer. His treatment approach includes the basic philosophy of including a variety of alternative treatments against cancer, with or without some concurrent therapies, including surgery, radiation, and chemotherapy. Dr. Schlachter's protocols usually include nutritional support, botanicals, detoxification methods, bio-oxidative therapies, hormonal balancing, homeopathic remedies, and acupuncture.

One of modern-day integrative medicine's "superstars" is **Dr. Stanislov Burzynski,** an immigrant from Poland who escaped communism, coming to the United States penniless in 1970. Dr. Burzynski's background includes a summa cum laude medical degree and a PhD in biochemistry—a rare academic achievement.

Like so many other serendipitous discoveries, Dr. Burzynski was originally studying protein chemistry in mushrooms, looking for a newer form of antibiotic. He quickly became an international expert in peptide chemistry, and in the course of his work he found that cancer patients were lacking certain inherent peptides that were present in noncancer patients.

Dr. Burzynski drew the correct conclusion that this deficiency of certain protein peptides might hold the clue to treating cancers by replacing the substances he called antineoplastons. When he first defected to the US from Poland in 1970, Dr. Burzynski's prestigious curriculum vitae secured him a research position at Baylor College of Medicine, in Houston, Texas, working with other distinguished peptide-oriented scientists.

Eventually, after battling the FDA for an IND (investigational new drug) application, Dr. Burzynski opened his own clinic in Houston in the late 1970s, which is world-renowned today and where he has, over the past thirty-three years, treated all forms of adult as well as many childhood cancers, all in Stage IV. Dr. Burzynski's work with advanced brain cancers has earned him access to an IND with the FDA, allowing patients to legally receive antineoplaston therapy.

His theory, in short, states that there is a system of peptide communication in the human body that parallels the immune system communications, and this system can inhibit the growth of cancer cells. The cancer cells that are missing antineoplaston are present in most cancer patients. Giving these peptides as replacement therapy can inhibit the growth of these cancers and cause remissions without toxicity to any normal cells in the body. In addition to his peptide treatments, Dr. Burzynski uses diet and supplement recommendations, as well as low-dose chemotherapy in most of his protocols.

Lastly, the groundbreaking enzyme therapy promoted by the late **Dr. William D. Kelley** in the 1960s and 1970s included the combination of high-dose supplements and pancreatic enzyme therapies. Dr. Kelley, a dentist by training, followed the teachings of embryologist Dr. John Beard from Scotland, who popularized the trophoblastic theory. This theory is based on the similarities between cancer cells and the trophoblastic cells of early pregnancy. Trophoblastic cells are the earliest differentiated cells following fertilization, which lead to the formation of the placenta and the umbilical cord.

Both cancer cells and trophoblastic cells produce a hormone called chorionic gonadotropin. These early cells are protected by a protein coating, and one of the major tenets of Dr. Kelley's enzyme therapy has been to remove the protein coat with pancreatic enzyme treatments and expose the cancer cell to immune system vulnerability. The rapid growth of the trophoblastic cell is compared to the invasive, rapid growth of a cancer cell in its prototypic philosophy. It is reported that Dr. Kelley even cured his own pancreatic cancer using his enzyme therapies and remained in remission for over 30 years.

Dr. Nicholas Gonzalez trained under Dr. Kelley as a medical student when he was at Cornell University. Dr. Gonzalez reviewed Dr. Kelley's data thoroughly and was so impressed that he changed his specialty interest to working with cancer patients in New York State, and today he is the most vocal practitioner following the Kelley Enzyme Therapy.

CHAPTER NINE

AN INTEGRATIVE VIEW OF CANCER PROMOTERS AND TRIGGERS

What are the major triggers or promoters of cancer from an integrative oncologist's point of view? Diet and lifestyle, along with many other triggers (which will be discussed later), have been identified as contributors.

All of these triggers first inflict injury to the DNA molecule, which is your genetic blueprint. Following this initial DNA injury there is a latent period of varying length; during this time various promoters are at work, which are designed to further steer the injured cell into a precancerous cell and ultimately, into a fully identifiable cancer cell.

The multiple promoters that contribute to the creation of

a cancer can be categorized into the following major classes, further described below: inherited disorders, physical/environmental factors, diet, infectious agents, toxic metals, and a miscellaneous class that includes pesticides, tobacco, and even some FDA-approved drugs.

INHERITED DISORDERS (MIASMS)

The first group is the inherited disorders. The integrative oncologist describes this group as miasms, a concept first presented by Samuel Hahnemann, the "father of homeopathy," in the early 1800s. Hahnemann described a miasm as an inherited predisposition to certain chronic diseases, including cancer.

Hahnemann's three major miasms included "psoric"—a predilection for cancer, diabetes, arthritis, and mental illnesses, including schizophrenia. The second miasm was "syphilitic," deriving from the residual inherited effects of the syphilitic bacterial infection. The third miasm according to Hahnemann was the "sycotic" miasm, arising from a family history of gonorrheal infections.

In the past fifty years, homeopathic physicians have added a cancer miasm, which is best described as a combination of all of the other three miasms.

Gene research over the past three decades has more clearly defined the genetic relationship to certain cancers. This research has determined that some cancers—including thyroid cancers, melanomas, and breast, ovarian, and colorectal cancers—run predictably along family lines. It has also identified mutations in certain genes that are directly related to the propensity to develop a single or group of cancers. As examples,

BRCA1 and BRCA2 relate to ovarian and breast cancers specifically.

It must be emphasized, however, that gene mutations account for no more than 5% of all cancers.

The concept of oncogenes, discovered in the 1970s, shed more light on the genetic origins of cancer. Oncogenes are altered genes that can transform normal cells into cancer cells. Genetic research has now concluded that cancers of the colon, lung, and pancreas can be triggered by mutations in oncogenes.

EXTERNAL PHYSICAL TRIGGERS FOR TURNING CELLS CANCEROUS

Numerous clinical studies have identified various physical factors as triggers for the transformation of a normal cell into either a precancerous or a cancerous cell. These include sunlight, for melanomas and other skin cancers, including squamous cell cancers and basal cell cancers.

The ultraviolet radiation from sunlight is the main trigger factor in more than 450,000 cases of skin cancers per year in the US. Ultraviolet radiation causes a mutation of the p-53 gene. The damaging effects of bad sunburns in youth may not manifest as skin cancer until decades later. These cancers typically develop in persons with fair skin and blue eyes who are of northern European extraction.

Another physical factor in the causation of cancer is exposure to electromagnetic fields, increasingly common due to the explosion in electronic technologies: cell phones, computers, television screens, iPods, electrical transmission poles, over-head lighting, and more. Epidemiological studies show that brain cancers, head and neck cancers, breast cancers, and various hematological cancers may be triggered by these invisible electromagnetic fields.

A closely aligned physical factor is geopathic stress, originating from magnetic sources in underground fractures in the earth's core and from underground water veins, which emit energy fields.

Yet another physical factor is radiation. There are three major sources of radiation triggers or initiators. One is nuclear radiation from nuclear plants or industrial sources. The second is ionizing radiation, which originates from X-rays taken in hospitals and outpatient radiation labs or from radiation therapy clinics. The third is radon gas, a radioactive, colorless, and odorless gas found in granite-containing soils in many areas of the country that have been listed as triggers for lung, gastric, colorectal, and hematologic malignancies.

Too much radiation exposure may be due in part to defensive medicine, or overzealous testing by clinicians of various specialties. As a consequence, it's becoming an increasingly serious matter in modern medicine where tort reform is going to be a necessity not only to reduce costs, but also to prevent patients from undergoing too much unnecessary testing. Tort reform would allow doctors to order fewer tests and diagnostic radiological procedures, putting the patient under less physical and mental stress.

For example, a single CAT scan of the chest may be equivalent to 100 plain chest X-ray films in terms of radiation exposure, and a PET scan performed with a radio-tagged sugar molecule may deliver five times the radiation dosage and exposure of a single CAT scan.

This overzealous testing is bombarding the patient with enormous amounts of radiation. This is self-defeating and serves only to weaken and suppress an already compromised immune system that must do battle with an increasing mass of cancer cells. Overexposure to radiation is essentially breaking down the front line of defense in the human body.

DIETARY CANCER TRIGGERS

Dietary and lifestyle choices, including the use of alcohol, tobacco, and hormonal medications, account for as many as 60% to 65% of all cancers, according to the National Academy of Sciences.

We integrative oncologists believe that the ideal diet for all cancer patients is a diet low in simple sugars, red meat, milk products, fried foods, cured or smoked meats, food additives, sodas, and saturated fats.

Of utmost importance is the elimination of simple sugars. Cancer cells have more insulin receptors than any other cells in the body and they thrive on simple sugars.

Cancer-fighting solid food preferences should include the use of colored vegetables, including peppers, squashes, melons, berries, and citrus fruits; organic foods should be consumed whenever possible, including organic range-grown fowl and farmed fish (free of mercury).

Along with poor dietary choices, we must include the cancer causative roles played by fluoridated and chlorinated water, and water polluted by heavy metals and toxic chemicals.

Cancer-fighting liquid preferences should include fresh juicing, green tea, berry juices and pomegranate juice, as well as pure/bottled waters, and especially waters that have been filtered to produce high alkaline content.

INFECTIOUS AGENTS CAN BE CANCER TRIGGERS

There is a long list of infectious agents that have been identified as triggers or promoters, or simply stated, as basic carcinogens.

One of the major bacterial promoters identified in the past thirty years is the H. pylori bacteria, which not only is the prime cause of peptic ulcer disease but also gastric carcinoma and distal esophageal cancers.

Major viral triggers include, first and foremost, the leading cause of the worldwide pandemic of hepatocellular (liver) cancer, known as the hepatitis B and C viruses.

The human papilloma virus, known as HPV types 16 and 18, has been identified as the major cause of female cervical cancer and is the only viral-causing cancer for which a vaccine is currently available.

Also, the Epstein-Barr virus, known as EBV, has been recognized as a causative agent in certain lymphomas, namely Burkitt's lymphoma, as well as in nasopharyngeal cancers and anogenital cancers.

A 2009 finding of a retroviral agent (XMRV) as the cause of chronic fatigue immune dysfunction syndrome may act as a causative agent in prostate cancer, chronic lymphocytic leukemia, and non-Hodgkin's lymphoma.

Kaposi's sarcoma is a rare form of skin cancer and has been associated with the human herpes virus number 8, so-called HHV-8. The relationship of herpes zoster virus and various cancers is undisputable; however, an exact causation remains unproven.

For the past fifty years certain parasitic infections have been known to be associated with specific cancers. These include *Schistosoma hematobium* and bladder cancer, and *Clonorchis sinensis* and liver cancer.

Toxoplasmosis has been described also as a causative parasitic agent for lymphomas, but a relationship has not been scientifically proven.

The human immunodeficiency virus, or HIV, which destroys the body's B cell population, has for the past thirty years been described as the major trigger for a number of various cancers, either directory or indirectly, including—most commonly—Hodgkin's and non-Hodgkin's lymphoma, Kaposi's sarcoma, primary central nervous system lymphomas, head and neck cancers, and anogenital cancers.

Systemic fungal infections have been associated with various organ cancers; however, proof of this relationship is still lacking. Chief among these infections are systemic candidiasis and aspergillosis organisms.

TOXIC METALS CAN BE CANCER TRIGGERS

Heavy metal toxicity can be easily detected by hair analysis, which is superior to blood and urine testing, and is routinely used by integrative oncologists, but rarely if ever checked for by conventional oncologists. These toxins are also a hidden trigger for cancer initiation, and many toxic metal alloys can be found in dental amalgams.

Swiss scientist Dr. Thomas Rau has proven that each tooth in the human body relates to a specific organ. In his research he has found that 90% of all breast cancer is associated with a dental disease specifically of the first upper molar/tooth on the same side. This tooth is referred to as the breast meridian.

Biological dentists have long known that there is a solid relationship between dental diseases and many systemic diseases, including cancer. A decayed or infected tooth, or a gum or root-canal infection, can block and disturb energy flow along specific acupuncture meridians, which in turn can adversely affect specific corresponding organ functioning.

Dental amalgams usually contain more than 50% mercury and lesser amounts of silver, tin, and nickel. A patient with a mouthful of silver fillings will often show toxic levels of all these heavy-metal toxins in hair analysis testing.

Heavy metals act as free radicals, which are highly charged reactive ions and can damage the DNA structure and trigger cancers.

Other heavy metals such as arsenic, uranium, lead, and cadmium are known carcinogens for various cancers including lung, skin, bladder, and bone marrow cancers, including leukemias, lymphomas, and myelomas. These metals are often introduced into the body via water supply or exposure to pesticides.

The only certain way of removing heavy-metal toxins from the body is by mobilizing them from deep tissues through the process of chelation therapy. Chelation, meaning "crablike," refers to the action of specific amino acids (EDTA, DMSA, etc.)

to solubilize the heavy metal and allow the metal ion to be excreted safely through the kidneys.

OTHER NOTABLE CANCER TRIGGERS

Herbicides and pesticides are a growing problem of enormous proportions. It is estimated that in 2010 more than 500 varieties of pesticides were approved by the FDA for use on food crops, and consequently ended up being consumed by humans.

The enormity of the problem cannot be overstated, as there has been a more than twelvefold increase in pesticide exposure within the past 70 years. What is even more frightening is even if these agents are banned in the US, the increased importation of fruits, vegetables, tea, and coffee from other countries without regulatory control end up on our dining room tables.

Tobacco is another notable trigger. A third of the United States adult population either smokes or uses smokeless tobacco, and another unknown percentage is exposed to passive smoke in confined spaces such as cars, buses, clubs, houses, apartments, workplaces, and theaters. It is no surprise, then, that tobacco remains the number one carcinogen in the US, according to a report by the US Public Health Service.

Lung cancer related to smoking is now the leading cause of cancer deaths in both men and women, and one of the most lethal and rapidly growing of all cancers. It is estimated that there are as many as 450,000 cases of cancers diagnosed yearly related to tobacco smoke. Approximately 150,000 deaths per year occur from lung cancer alone.

In addition to head and neck cancers, including cancers of the salivary glands, sinuses, and nasopharyngeal areas, tobacco smoke can either trigger or promote cancer of the tongue, tonsils, larynx, trachea, bronchial tubes, and the lung itself.

Cancers of the esophagus, stomach, pancreas, kidneys, cervix, and bladder have also been connected with tobacco smoke.

Smokeless tobacco has been proven to be both a trigger and promoter of lip, tongue, oral mucous membrane, and tonsillar carcinomas.

At autopsy, in my years as a pathologist, I was well aware that the lungs of a smoker are laced with and permeated with varying sized black-tar residue, giving the appearance of an overused air filter on an automobile engine. This compares to a pink, sponge-like appearance at autopsy from the lung of a child or an adult nonsmoker.

Often described as a co-carcinogen along with tobacco is alcohol. In excess, alcohol is an initiator or promoter of cancers of the head and neck, esophagus, stomach, liver, pancreas, and bladder.

Long-term use of alcohol can also result in cirrhosis and excessive iron loading in the liver, a condition called hemosiderosis. This condition reduces natural killer cell function and is immunosuppressive. Both of these factors contribute to create an ideal setting for cancer initiation.

There is evidence that FDA-approved drugs themselves may account for as many as 250,000 to 300,000 deaths per year in the US, a figure translating to somewhere between the sixth to eighth leading cause of death in adults in the United States. More frightening is the fact that this number is under-reported.

You only need to listen to the disclaimers in Big Pharma's commercials on the radio and television to learn that some approved drugs are actually initiators or promoters of cancer, as admitted by the FDA.

It is well-documented in the Stanford University Medical Center report on the long-term effects of chemotherapy, based on their Hodgkin's disease patients who had received multiple drug chemotherapy, that there is as high as a 3% to 5% increase of subsequent cancers, including leukemias and sarcomas.

If you combine poor diet and nutritional habits with poor lifestyle choices, especially tobacco use, abuse of alcohol, and sexual habits (which can be triggers for HIV and HPV), one realizes that close to 70% of all cancers can be accounted for by these factors alone. The remaining 30% is made up of all the other causes mentioned in this chapter. Severe stress and toxic emotions probably contribute another 5% to this latter figure, but these are factors almost impossible to measure.

CHAPTER TEN

THE ART OF CHOOSING DRUGS AND SUPPLEMENTS

Conventional oncology maintains a vast arsenal of both old and new drugs to consider for each individual patient prior to deciding upon the best drug protocol. Will it be a single drug, two drugs, or multiple drug chemotherapy? At one point in the late 1970s and early 1980s, there was actually a drug protocol written by the Northern California Oncology Group (NCOG) for small-cell carcinoma of the lung that contained twelve different chemotherapy agents given on a rotating basis. The outcome of this study was dismal and resulted in shortened overall survival for patients and significant multi-organ toxicity.

While most independent and well-meaning oncologists base their therapeutic decisions for first-, second-, or third-line chemo drug protocols on the results of the latest published studies, or on the yearly presentations given at the prestigious American Society of Clinical Oncology meeting, often it is akin to entering a dark room with a handful of darts and hoping to hit the center of the dartboard. Different lines of chemo are often prescribed for patients if they become resistant to the first one they're using, or it simply doesn't work for their type of cancer.

Without knowledge of the genetic markers for specific tumors to guide them in composing an effective chemo drug protocol, an oncologist is truly "shooting in the dark."

It's important for cancer patients to know that there are no chemotherapy protocols that demonstrate 100% efficacy. Basing drug selection on clinical studies that show anywhere from 40% to 70% or even 80% response rates is still only, at best, guesswork that turns cancer patients into virtual guinea pigs.

In fact, most multidrug studies using more than two agents is almost always "off-label" usage since Big Pharma doesn't normally study more than two drugs at a time, and hence the term "evidence-based medicine" used by conventional oncology is meaningless because of these factors. In this instance, off-label means any drug that is used for a condition not directly related to its stated usage directions.

The integrative oncologist dramatically parts company with conventional oncology by presenting the patient with options that empower him or her to take an active role in deciding what he or she wants to happen to their bodies. These five options are as follows:

1. Strict protocol chemotherapy based upon results of chemosensitivity testing
2. Low-dose fractionated chemotherapy, either alone or with insulin potentiation
3. Either #1 or #2 above with complementary therapies based on supplement testing for genetic markers
4. Complementary therapy alone following chemosensitivity testing
5. Supportive therapy for patients who are too far advanced for any other type of treatment

A core component of this decision-making by the patient and integrative practitioner is the chemosensitivity test. This process begins with a portion of the cancerous tissue, which amounts to either one gram or more taken from a solid tumor mass. This could come from breast tissue, lung tissue, colorectal tissue, sarcoma tissue, or from the blood of a leukemic patient.

"All or nothing" chemotherapy based on statistical extrapolation was the only option for patients until the early 1990s, when medical oncologist Robert A. Nagourney developed a chemosensitivity test called the Ex-Vivo Apoptotic Assay.

As director of the Rational Therapeutics Laboratory in Long Beach, California, Dr. Nagourney developed the previously unrecognized concept that "it is not that cancer cells grow too much but rather that they die too little." For forty years prior to this point, the entire cancer research industry was focused on cancer as being a disease of uncontrolled cell proliferation, with the cancer cells remaining "immortal" until the host, meaning the patient, died.

Dr. Nagourney's test can determine the likelihood of more than a hundred chemotherapy agents, given singly or in doublets, to cause a cancer cell to go into apoptosis, or programmed cell death. By culturing the living cancer cells with various chemotherapy agents, Dr. Nagourney has shown that the oncologist can tailor-make a protocol of a successful drug or drugs to benefit each individual patient.

His results routinely yield a two- to threefold increase in success rates over blindly given chemotherapy protocols. Despite these successes, this test is still not widely used by conventional oncologists in the US today.

There are several limitations with Dr. Nagourney's test. First is the requirement for an actual portion of the cancer mass to be removed, preserved, and tested. If cancer tissue is in the brain, lungs, liver, bones, or deep in the pancreatic tissues, removing a sufficient amount of tissue for testing is not only difficult and risky to the patient's health, but may require a major surgical procedure.

The second problem with the Nagourney test concerns the very important and comprehensive determination of which supplements will be effective and useful complementary therapy for treating the cancer patient. This limitation is addressed by two other tests that have emerged in the past ten years—a test from German cancer laboratory Biofocus that involves whole blood harvesting of cancer cells and a Greek test developed by the Research Genetic Cancer Centre (RGCC) that also tests cancer genes for mutations and routinely evaluates and scores the efficacy of thirty-eight different herbs, vitamins, and minerals as well as such varied treatments as hydrogen peroxide and hyperthermia.

The chemosensitivity testing methodology from Biofocus includes the following:

1. Isolation from sample of cancer cells and the development of primary cultures
2. Each culture includes in the cultivation media a cytostatic drug (a drug that prevents cancer cells from multiplying rather than killing them)
3. Testing of genes by micro-array analysis, which become targets for cytostatics, or they are involved in resistance phenotype, or in the metastatic procedure
4. Verification of the analysis by small-scale viability testing of the cultures

The Greek RGCC testing laboratory involves probes for the following genes:

1. TS
2. DHFR
3. Tubulin
4. Topoisomerase
5. SHMT
6. DPD
7. IP
8. p27
9. p53
10. DNA
11. Methyltransferase
12. 06 acyltransferase
13. DNA deaminase
14. MPP
15. LRP
16. GST
17. BEGF
18. PDGF
19. EGF
20. TGFb
21. MMP9
22. Nucleotide reductase
23. Cox-2
24. S-lox
25. SS-r
26. C-erb2

It isn't within the scope of this book to detail the highly complex biochemical analysis of all of these genetic factors and their relationships to existing chemotherapy and targeted agents. Suffice it to say, however, with these results in hand, the integrative oncologist can now furnish each patient with a definitive blueprint of which agents will work best for his or her specific cancer genetics.

The Greek and German tests also furnish extremely helpful information to the integrative oncologist, based on analysis, with respect to the following supplements:

- artemisia
- hydrogen peroxide
- ascorbic acid
- vitamin B6
- mistletoe
- ukrain
- vitamin B17
- colloidal silver
- indol-3 carbinol
- C-statin
- Poly-MVA
- thalidomide
- quercetin
- COX-2
- cytokines
- Carnivora
- coenzyme Q-10 (CoQ-10)
- Essiac tea
- modified citrus pectin
- IP-6

- pancreatic enzymes
- salvestrol
- Uncaria tomentosa
- noni juice
- acetogenins
- cesium chloride
- maitake
- curcumin
- green tea extract
- melatonin
- ellagic acid
- L-methionine
- N-acetyl cysteine
- vitamin B3
- L-carnitine
- vitamin E
- superoxide dismutase
- selenium
- aloe vera
- alpha interferon

The newly opened Goodgene lab in Texas also offers comprehensive testing.

With this valuable information in hand, the next step for the integrative oncologist is to review the data and then compose and assign to the patient a definitive protocol, taking into consideration the patient's choice of options, prior therapies, and the least toxic and most effective drug or drugs recommended, along with the recommended supplements based on testing.

There is no greater support an oncologist can give his or her patient than this thorough, scientific, evidence-based blueprint. As for the duration of treatment, this is determined by either complete remission, which means disappearance of all measurable disease, or the progression of disease, in which case another agent or agents would be utilized.

Like everything else in medicine, there are no absolutes and the integrative oncologist's judgment comes into play significantly in the production of the treatment protocol. This, in reality, is the essence of the art of medicine.

HOW MUCH SUPPLEMENTATION IS ENOUGH?

As mentioned, a major difference between conventional and integrative oncology concerns the use of vitamin and mineral supplements in bolstering the immune system to help treat cancer.

This philosophical difference about treatment is exacerbated by policies of the US Food and Drug Administration and its nutritional regulatory branches, which publish recommended daily allowances, or RDAs, of specific vitamins and minerals. By law, through a required packaging and labeling process, manufacturers and distributors of foods, vitamins, and minerals must specify the percentage of these substances that each particular product contains.

However, on all of these product labels, from cereal boxes to milk cartons, the term "100%" refers to the least amount of a vitamin or mineral that the FDA, through its physician panels, deems necessary to maintain good health. In other words, these minimum levels are the absolute lowest amounts necessary to prevent deficiency diseases such as scurvy, rickets, pellagra, beriberi, and pernicious anemia, to name the more common ones.

When these standards were developed in the late 1940s and early 1950s, vitamin and mineral testing procedures were limited by the technology of that period, whereas the modern equipment of today gives much more accurate and meaningful results.

These archaic RDA levels continue to be recognized as the "gold standard" by the FDA, though they fail to meet the true demands of the human body, especially amidst the increased onslaught of serious cancers, severe cardiovascular disease and strokes, environmental toxins and pollutants, chemotherapy drugs, and virulent viral, bacterial, and parasitic diseases.

The RDA for vitamins and minerals can vary significantly from the *optimal* daily allowances. For instance:

Vitamin C: The RDA is only 60 mg per day compared to an optimal daily allowance of 1,000 mg per day. Dr. Linus Pauling, who won the Nobel Prize for his work in vitamin C research, was purported to take up to 19 grams of vitamin C daily and he lived until his mid-nineties, staying active on the lecture circuit up until his death.

Vitamin A: The RDA is 1,000 mcg per day, and yet the optimal daily allowance is believed to be somewhere between 15,000 and 25,000 IU per day.

Vitamin D3: Now widely used in all cancer cases, but especially in prostate cancer, breast cancer, colorectal cancer, and lymphomas, vitamin D3 has an RDA of only 400 IU per day, and yet most alternative physicians would like to see vitamin D3 in the range of 80 to 100, and this usually requires between 5,000 to 15,000 IU per day.

Vitamin E: The RDA is only 30 IU per day, yet it is recommended that patients with severe dementias receive doses in the range of 1,600 IU per day.

Through these examples you can see the huge discrepancy that exists between the outdated RDAs—which are endorsed by conventional mainstream medicine—and the optimal daily doses recommended by most integrative and alternative physicians.

CHAPTER ELEVEN

A KINDER, GENTLER FORM OF CHEMOTHERAPY

It is the knee-jerk tendency of conventional oncologists to use full-dose, heavy-duty chemotherapy out of the starting gate to treat their cancer patients. This is done without respect to the severe toxicities that may occur as soon as after the first dose, such as cytopenias, otherwise referred to as severe bone marrow depression.

After almost forty years of practicing cancer medicine, both as a straight-line conventional oncologist and for the past fifteen years as an integrative oncologist, I have come to see every horrible type of toxicity imaginable when this conventional oncology approach is taken. It's not unusual for patients to end up hospitalized with severe white-blood-cell depression and sepsis or pneumonia simply because their bodies couldn't handle the full dose of chemotherapy.

Yes, even death can occur after one cycle of full-dose chemotherapy!

The conventional oncologist's main hope is that the chemotherapy will kill the cancer before it kills the patient.

There are many examples of drugs on the market that initially were dosed too high, and only after intolerable toxicities were witnessed was the dosage reduced to fractionated levels, or given at lower doses on a more frequent basis. The drug might be given intravenously in weekly increments for three weeks out of the month, for example, rather than in full dose every three to four weeks.

This was the case for a number of agents, including the taxane family of drugs, the topotecans, Mitomycin-C, etoposide, and the platinum-based family of drugs, including cisplatin, carboplatin, and oxaliplatin.

In the case of the taxanes, the most common approach recommended today in breast cancer is to give the drug at a lower weekly dose, three out of four weeks per month, instead of a dose three times higher every twenty-one days, as was done when the drug was first prescribed for patients. Many fewer side effects are generated this way.

Many integrative cancer centers in the US today will often divide a dosage into daily or every-other-day doses, two or three times a week, in order to mitigate what would otherwise be severe toxicities.

This kinder, gentler form of chemotherapy has come to be labeled insulin potentiated targeted low-dose therapy. The therapy almost always reduces or diminishes the toxic side-effects of conventional chemotherapy.

Insulin potentiated therapy, often referred to as IPT, dates back to the late 1940s and was developed by Dr. Donato Perez Garcia in South America. Because of a paucity of clinical trials using IPT, the FDA considers this method of treatment "off-label."

It's important for patients to keep in mind that the pharmaceutical "bible" of medical drugs, the *Physician's Desk Reference* (PDR), which is updated yearly, allows any licensed physician in any state to prescribe drugs from this resource in an off-label fashion. Also, anytime a patient is undergoing a second-, third-, or fourth-line protocol, this treatment is by definition off-label, as no clinical studies are available to verify its efficacy. What this means is that if you are doing a second or third round of chemotherapy with a new drug, there have been no studies done to prove how effective that drug will be in treating you.

The many advantages of insulin potentiated therapy include:

* It has been successfully used in cancer treatments since the late 1940s.
* It targets the cancer cell without destroying normally dividing cells.
* Because it vectors in on cancer cells specifically, very low doses of between 10% and 20% can be used effectively.
* It spares vital organs and especially bone marrow cells, including red blood cells, white blood cells, and platelets.
* It has been shown to be minimally suppressive to the immune system.

◆ Common chemotherapy related side effects such as
chemo brain, nausea, vomiting, diarrhea, rashes, hair
loss, or severe fatigue are rare with insulin potentiated
therapy.

With all of these advantages, one has to ask why Big Pharma
and the FDA don't pursue clinical studies on this methodology.
The likely answer is that Big Pharma would lose money if all
oncologists cut their drug dosing by 90%, thus lowering costs
to patients, insurers, and the overall health-care system.

IPT is a procedure for administering conventional/FDA-
approved chemotherapy drugs "off-label" in conjunction with
insulin and in fractionated low doses directly into cancer cells,
unlike conventional chemotherapy, which poisons both the
good and bad cells in the body. The theory behind the mecha-
nism of IPT is based on the fact that cancer cells have many
more insulin receptors on the cell surface than all other cells
in the body. Because of this, small doses of insulin "trick" the
cancer cell into being more receptive to the chemotherapy
molecule and, therefore, lower doses are required.

Additionally, with IPT, chemotherapy is delivered through
the IV at the height of cancer cell stimulation and is avidly
taken up by the cancer cell. Essentially, this delivery system
works like a smart bomb or Trojan horse.

The dismal and discouraging overall survival rates of just
2.1% in the US over a five-year period for Stage IV adult cancer
patients, as reported in conventional oncology's own literature,
should be reason enough to explore alternative, safer, cheaper,
and more effective treatment protocols.

CHAPTER TWELVE

WHAT INTEGRATIVE ONCOLOGY PATIENTS SAY

When fifty-seven-year-old Carol reached a dead end with the treatment options that oncologists in Ohio offered her for Stage IV colon cancer, she knew that she had to find her own way back to good health. She happened to read Suzanne Somers' book, *Knockout,* with its chapter on me and Century Wellness in Reno, and decided to try our integrative approach to fighting her cancer.

"My doctors back home had run out of options for me," she explained in a 2010 recording posted on YouTube. "I had gone through twelve rounds of chemotherapy for colon cancer.

Then I was diagnosed with ovarian cancer and went through six more chemo treatments. When my Stage IV colon cancer metastasized to my liver and lungs, they gave me another twelve chemo sessions, which was really hard on my body. Then they told me I only had six to twelve months of life left. I thought to myself, this is crazy. There has to be a better way."

Accompanied by her daughter, Ariel, who works in the medical field, Carol traveled to Reno and spent several weeks at our clinic. One of the first things we did was to give her a chemosensitivity test to determine which chemo drugs were effective for her type of cancer.

Here the daughter, Ariel, picks up her mother's story: "We were skeptical when we first came here because our doctors had given a hopeless diagnosis. You may be thinking, 'My oncologist did send my blood out and figured out what kind of cancer I have.' What they do traditionally is send your blood out and the therapy they give you is based on clinical trials that work for most people. For colon cancer you would receive the same treatment in Ohio that you would in Tennessee. What oncologists don't tell you is that in other countries, such as Germany, where Dr. Forsythe sends your blood, they actually examine your blood so you can find out exactly what drug is compatible for your exact type of colon cancer."

Carol then added, "What I found out is that most every chemo drug I was given is really not that effective for the type of cancer I have. Now with the lower doses of chemo that I do take, it's effective, there are fewer side effects, and I feel great. My energy level is back and I work full time again at a college in Ohio. My last PET scan showed no new lesions or tumors and no growth in the cancer. I am not supposed to be alive and feel as healthy as I do. When your doctor says there is nothing left that we can do, don't believe them. There is always something else out there."

As I indicated in my introduction to this book, when an oncologist begins telling you to "get your affairs in order" and "check out hospice care," that physician has given up on you, which no practitioner should ever do. It is these hard-to-treat patients who might benefit most from an integrative approach to cancer care. A good example is David, a sixty-four-year-old man from Sacramento with advanced Stage IV colon/rectal cancer. He had been told to enter a hospice program but he wasn't willing to give up on life, so he came to Century Wellness instead. We discovered the chemo drugs he had been on weren't effective. Once we got him on the right drugs and supplements, his cancer cleared up. Today he lives an active life and plays golf two or three times a week.

Barbara of Yakima, Washington, had a similar experience with her Stage IV lung cancer. "I was told by my oncologist to go to a hospice. But I didn't want to sit around waiting for death, so my husband of fifty-three years of marriage called Century Wellness. Despair was changed to hope. I discovered that we have a power within us that can heal. We have to give it the help we need."

By empowering our own immune system to harness its natural resources to aid in the fight against cancer, we employ the most powerful weapon we have to bring back a state of wellness. Integrative oncology's emphasis on fortifying the immune system with a proper diet and supplements often surprises cancer patients who are used to being told by conventional oncologists that diet doesn't really matter, only drugs and radiation do.

"It has been such an eye-opener to learn about the role of our immune system and the need to focus on our diet," observes David, a fifty-seven-year-old from Columbia, South Carolina, with prostate cancer, who came to Century Wellness with his wife, Debbie, who worked as a registered nurse. "No one back home had ever told us about the importance of the immune system and healthy foods we should be eating to help fight cancer. We also get psychological and spiritual support here that I never found from physicians before. We have been given new hope."

Bret is a forty-six-year-old lawyer from Los Altos, California, whose Stage III brain tumor couldn't completely be removed during surgery because of the tumor's location. "The surgeon had to leave part of the tumor in my brain to protect my motor functions. It could still proliferate and kill me. It actually does kill most people. After surgery I went through a scary process of radiation and chemotherapy, which I wish I hadn't done because the tumor remained there. I came to Century Wellness for three weeks with my wife and child. The clinic gave me painless treatments of supplements, Poly-NVA, and intravenous fluids. It's now been over a year and I'm fine. Not only that, but my entire treatment team at UC San Francisco, where I had the surgery, is amazed because the tumor was gone in my most recent MRI. My advice if you have cancer is to run, not walk, to Century Wellness."

In contrast to conventional slash-and-burn approaches to cancer treatment, with its focus on just that part of the body that is diseased, integrative oncologists seek to address the health needs of the entire human being. Our philosophy is that we want to remove the causes of cancer as we treat the entire body to rid it of disease. We also want to prevent the cancer's recurrence.

Mary Kathryn, a fifty-one-year-old mother of two from Chicago diagnosed with thyroid cancer, makes this point eloquently. "Since I've been here (at Century Wellness), in the rooms where we get our IV infusions, our chairs are just a few feet apart. We patients talk a lot. We laugh and network. I've been in a regular hospital setting and you don't get that. It's a really holistic care approach here."

"Once I got here," Mary Kathryn continues, "I found out that I probably had my cancer for a decade. It was slow growing. (At Century Wellness) they said, 'We'll make your body healthy so your cancer will go away.' They got rid of toxins in my body. They treated my mind. They treated my entire body to get rid of the cause of cancer, not just the nodule in my throat. That's why I came here and that's what is happening."

To view YouTube testimonials by many of the cancer patients mentioned in this chapter, along with others, go to: http://www.youtube.com/user/hopehealinglife.

RESULTS AFFIRM THE INTEGRATIVE PROCESS

The implementation of the Forsythe Immune Therapy (FIT) protocol, the proprietary treatment we use at the Century Wellness Clinic, in Stage IV adult cancers has shown outcome-based study results that have outshined conventional five-year results from conventional chemotherapy.

More importantly, these results are achieved without the multiple corresponding adverse toxicities that accompany toxic full-dose conventional chemotherapy. These integrative results leave the patient's immune system and organ function undamaged and still able to fight off challenges from bacterial, viral, and parasitic infections. Our patients, for the most part, do not suffer from hair loss, nausea, vomiting, diarrhea, or debilitating nerve damage.

FIT protocol patients receive supplements to strengthen and fortify the body's own immune function and allow for self-healing. These procedures provide a hostile internal environment for cancer cells, harming their ability to proliferate. Depriving cancer cells of their most basic nutritional requirement, namely simple sugars, is of paramount importance in every patient's war chest of battle plans.

Another important aspect of the FIT program is attempting to uncover the trigger or triggers of the underlying malignant process. For example, the use of hair analysis to uncover toxic heavy metal overloading, especially with known carcinogens such as arsenic, cadmium, mercury, uranium, lead, and antimony, is vital as a first step to stripping them from the body through chelation therapies, which are given either intravenously, orally, or via rectal suppositories. Discovering chemical, infectious, and dental problems through electrodermal testing is another vital component in the toolbox of integrative oncology in general and in the FIT protocol specifically.

Detoxification with bio-oxidative therapies and high-dose vitamin C, combined with immune stimulating IVs, is vital to restoring the body's ability to successfully ward off the invading cancerous tissues.

When conventional oncology tells patients, "There is no cure for Stage IV cancers," they are clearly expressing their ignorance of the results of comprehensive integrative therapies such as the FIT protocol.

The following pages summarize a number of actual cases,

treated at the Century Wellness Clinic in Reno in the latest five-year, 500-patient study, and show how cancer cures and successful remissions can be obtained using thoughtful, patient-oriented, whole body, integrative oncology procedures.

Keep in mind that a probable cure is always measured as an equation of complete remission plus a given amount of time (usually at least five years). However, as mentioned earlier in this book, some cancers may lay dormant for many years and resurface when the immune system is injured through accident or trauma, surgical procedures, severe illness, or emotional trauma.

The following cases are arranged in order of longest time in remission to the most recent cases—with no remission being shorter than 18 months. To comply with medical privacy regulations, since the patients have not yet volunteered the use of their full names, only the patients' initials are used to identify each case. Each patient's type of cancer is highlighted in bold.

CASE #1—R.T.

A postmenopausal, white female from Wyoming in her mid-fifties with an original **Stage II breast cancer** has gone more than six years in complete remission using the FIT protocol. This Wyoming rancher developed metastases to her chest wall and has steadfastly refused all conventional chemotherapy and hormonal therapy treatments, nor has she had any radiation therapy.

CASE #2—S.W.

An active white female from Arizona in her late seventies with a six-year history of **metastatic breast cancer** with involvement of liver tumors, who refused conventional adjuvant chemotherapy and is enjoying an excellent stable remission. She visits our clinic every four to six months for IV therapy along with her oral FIT protocol. She has had low-dose, intermittent, mild oral chemotherapy. At the present time she shows no progression of disease and she actively plays tennis three times a week.

CASE #3—I.D.

A fifty-five-year-old black female from California with **Stage IV ovarian cancer**, diagnosed six years earlier and treated initially with standard protocol chemotherapy, which failed after she developed lung and mediastinal metastases. She was originally seen by me four years ago with advanced Stage IV disease. She was placed on the FIT protocol and currently is free of all disease, a complete remission, and she has not had any further chemotherapy or radiation therapy.

CASE #4—C.C.

A seventy-one-year-old white female from Miami with advanced **Stage IV esophageal carcinoma**, with proven metastases to the liver and mediastinum. She has been on the FIT protocol and visits our clinic two to three times per year for booster treatments. She has been in complete remission for the past five-and-a-half years and has required no further protocol chemotherapy or low-dose chemotherapy, nor any radiation therapy. She is free of pain. She has no difficulty swallowing, and her weight has been stable. Her performance level is at 100%.

CASE #5—E.U.

A sixty-two-year-old white female from Washington with **Stage IV carcinoma of the ovary** for more than five years. The patient was initially placed on the FIT protocol with low-dose intermittent oral chemotherapy. Her ascites (abdominal fluid) completely cleared up and her CA-125 cancer marker remains within the normal range. She has a 100% performance level and is in complete remission.

CASE #6—E.D.

A seventy-four-year-old white male from Nevada with a **soft tissue sarcoma** in his left groin with pelvic metastases who was treated with low-dose chemotherapy along with the FIT protocol. He has not had any recurrence of his metastatic disease and remains disease-free after a four-and-a-half-year period.

CASE #7—P.F.

A sixty-eight-year-old white male from California with **Stage IV metastatic carcinoma of the prostate** with pelvic and bony metastases. This patient is in a stable remission with a low prostate-specific antigen (PSA) level. He is asymptomatic, without bone pain or weight loss, and he has a performance status of 100%.

CASE #8—P.N.

A forty-eight-year-old white male with **Stage IV cancer of the appendix**, associated with a gelatinous peritoneal fluid accumulation. This patient is five years post-diagnosis and has stable/nonprogressive disease on the FIT protocol. His performance status is now 90%.

CASE #9—J.S.

A twenty-four-year-old white female from southern California with **Stage IV Hodgkin's disease** in her lungs, mediastinum, and pelvis, who is now more than four years in stable remission. She refused initial conventional chemotherapy and radiation, and she has been on the FIT protocol since first seeing me four years earlier. She has regression of her metastatic disease and is in a stable remission. She even underwent a successful full-term pregnancy during this period of time.

CASE #10—G.T.

A sixty-six-year-old white male from Bend, Oregon, with **metastatic prostate cancer** with metastatic disease to his lower spine, causing initial paraplegia of the lower extremities. The patient had initial radiation therapy to his lower back but refused conventional chemotherapy. He has been on intermittent hormonal therapy for the first two years but has now been stable for the past four years, with a normal PSA level and no neurologic loss in his lower extremities. His performance status is 100%.

CASE #11—W.G.:

A seventy-five-year-old white male from Vallejo, California, with **Stage IV prostate cancer**, diagnosed four years ago with bony metastases, who refused hormonal therapy, surgery, and radiation therapy. His PSA is now stable. He is asymptomatic. He has been on the FIT protocol for the past three-and-a-half years, and he has a 100% performance status.

CASE #12—R.W.

A sixty-three-year-old white female from Las Vegas with **metastatic Stage IV breast cancer** for the past four years, who has been on the FIT protocol, without chemotherapy or radiation therapy. Her bone metastases have resolved. Her tumor markers are in the normal range and she remains on the FIT protocol with a 100% performance status.

CASE #13—G.K.

A sixty-one-year-old white male from Idaho with **metastatic prostate cancer**, with pelvic and bony metastases, who has had radiation therapy to his lower spine and pelvis. The patient refused surgery. He has been on insulin potentiated therapy along with the FIT protocol, and he has stable, nonprogressive disease after three-and-a-half years, with an 80% performance status.

CASE #14—D.S.

A sixty-four-year-old white male from California with **Stage IV colorectal cancer**, with metastases to his liver. The patient was diagnosed four years ago and underwent conventional chemotherapy, which failed. He subsequently demonstrated progressive liver metastases. He was told to go on hospice care but instead the patient came to the Century Wellness Clinic, where he has been on the FIT protocol for the past two-and-a-half years. He is in complete remission and plays golf two to three times per week with a 100% performance status.

CASE #15—J.W.

A forty-two-year-old black male from Texas with **Stage IV Hodgkin's disease** for the past three years, with pulmonary and mediastinal metastases, along with bulky left chest wall and left axillary metastases. This patient from Houston refused standard Hodgkin's disease protocol chemotherapy or radiation therapy. He has been on the FIT protocol with low-dose insulin potentiated therapy and he currently has stable disease with a 90% performance status.

CASE #16—M.P.:

A forty-seven-year-old female from Colorado with **Stage IV anal cancer**, with metastases to her pelvis and inguinal lymph nodes with Stage IV disease. The patient refused surgery, colostomy, radiation, or standard chemotherapy three-and-a-half years ago. She is now on low-dose oral chemotherapy and on the FIT protocol, and she is enjoying complete remission with a 100% performance status.

CASE #17—A.A.

A twenty-four-year-old white female from Nevada with **Stage IV non-Hodgkin's lymphoma**, diagnosed four years ago with primary bone metastases to her right shoulder and right hip as well as her rib cage. She refused standard chemotherapy or radiation therapy. She was started on the FIT protocol three years ago and is now in a stable, complete remission with normal tumor markers. She was previously wheelchair-reliant and now is able to ambulate using either a cane or a walker. Her performance status is 90%.

CASE #18—J.T.

A twenty-eight-year-old white male from California with **Stage IV colorectal cancer** with liver metastases, diagnosed four years ago. He took standard chemotherapy for less than three months, when his disease progressed. At that time he decided that he only wanted alternative therapy and was started on the FIT protocol. He remains in a stable remission with a normal performance status of 100% and normal tumor markers, and he has not had any further conventional chemotherapy.

CASE #19—M.B.

A fifty-four-year-old white male from California with **Stage IV colorectal cancer** with metastases to his lungs and liver, diagnosed three-and-a-half years ago. The patient underwent standard chemotherapy for six months and then refused further chemotherapy. He was started on the FIT protocol two-and-a-half years ago and he is now in a stable remission, with a normal performance status of 100%.

CASE #20—T.T.

A sixty-seven-year-old white male from Arizona with **Stage IV malignant melanoma** with lung metastases. He was diagnosed four years ago but refused standard chemotherapy. He also refused a bone marrow transplant. The patient was started on the FIT protocol with low-dose insulin potentiated therapy, and he is now in a stable remission with a normal performance status of 100%.

CASE #21—J.S.

A fifty-one-year-old white male from Florida with **multiple myeloma**, diagnosed three-and-a-half years ago, associated with renal failure and bone metastases. The patient refused standard chemotherapy. He was started on the FIT protocol two-and-a-half years ago, along with low-dose insulin potentiated therapy. He is now in a stable remission with a 100% performance status.

CASE #22—R.F.

A sixty-four-year-old white male from Nevada with **a primary central nervous system lymphoma**, diagnosed three years ago. He was treated with whole brain radiation therapy and he had a previous left-sided hemiplegia which is now 90% resolved. He is now in complete remission with normal tumor markers, and he continues on the FIT protocol.

CASE #23—G.F.

A forty-four-year-old white male from Nevada with **Stage IV melanoma** with lung metastases, with metastases to his bilateral cervical lymph nodes. The patient refused initial chemotherapy. He started on the FIT protocol three years ago and he is now in a stable disease remission, with a 90% performance status.

CASE #24—R.S.

A sixty-two-year-old white male from Virginia with two separate cancers—a **primary cancer of the pancreas** and a **primary non-Hodgkin's lymphoma** involving his testes. The patient was diagnosed two years ago and started on the FIT protocol, along with low-dose insulin potentiated therapy. He is in a stable disease status with an 80% performance level.

CASE #25—M.B.

A seventy-four-year-old white female from California with **metastatic non-small-cell lung cancer**, diagnosed two years ago, with metastases to her liver, brain, and spine. The patient refused standard chemotherapy or radiation therapy. She was placed on the FIT protocol and low-dose insulin potentiated therapy. She is now in a stable disease remission.

Case #26—R.L.

A fifty-eight-year-old white male with **metastatic colorectal cancer**, with lung and liver metastases, diagnosed three years ago. He was treated with chemotherapy and after eighteen months his disease progressed. He refused further conventional therapy. He was placed on the FIT protocol with low-dose insulin potentiated therapy, and he is now in a stable disease status with a performance level of 90%.

CASE #27—M.N.

A forty-six-year-old white female college professor with **metastatic thyroid cancer**, with pulmonary metastases, diagnosed three-and-a-half years ago. The patient was treated with radio-iodine, which did not halt the progression of the disease in her lungs and in her cervical lymph nodes. She was started on the FIT protocol two years ago and is now in a stable disease status, without further progression of her metastatic disease. Her performance level is 90%.

CASE #28—L.D.

A forty-five-year-old white female from California with **Stage IV metastatic breast cancer**, diagnosed three years ago, with metastases to her lungs and bones. The patient had a short course of standard chemotherapy. Her disease progressed and she refused further conventional therapy. She then was started on the FIT protocol two years ago and she is now in complete remission, with normal tumor markers and a 100% performance level.

CASE #29—B.B.

A 44-year-old white male from California with **primary anaplastic astrocytoma** of the right brain, initially treated with surgery and radiation therapy. He refused chemotherapy and the patient had residual disease after completion of his radiation therapy. He was started on the FIT protocol, where all of his re-maining disease was treated and subsequently disappeared. He now has a 100% performance status without any neurological disabilities whatsoever.

CASE #30—S.W.

This forty-six-year-old white female from North Carolina was di-agnosed with **Stage IV non-small-cell lung cancer** two-and-a-half years ago. She received standard chemotherapy with a platinum-containing drug, but after six months her tumor progressed. She came to the Century Wellness Clinic and was placed on the FIT protocol. Her routine workup showed her to have platinum toxicity from her previous chemotherapy, and her chemosensi-tivity testing showed that two out of the three drugs she previ-ously received were ineffective for treatment of her cancer. She has since been maintained on low-dose oral chemotherapy and has been in a sustained remission for the past eighteen months with a 100% performance status.

CASE #31—T.C.

This fifty-one-year-old white female from Canada was diagnosed with **Stage IV non-small-cell lung cancer** two-and-a-half years ago. She has documented bone metastases and received che-motherapy while in Canada. However, her disease progressed and she came to the Century Wellness Clinic for alternative therapy. For the past year-and-a-half she has been in excellent remission, primarily on oral supplements, dietary control, and alkalinization. She has a 100% performance status and has had no progression in her disease.

CASE #32—K.P.

This sixty-two-year-old white female from Washington was diagnosed two-and-a-half years ago with **Stage IV renal cell carcinoma**, with pulmonary metastases. She underwent chemosensitivity testing and was subsequently placed on low-dose insulin potentiated therapy along with the FIT protocol. She has remained in stable remission for the past year-and-a-half, with an excellent performance status of 100%.

CASE #33—J.R.

A sixty-three-year-old white male from California with **head and neck cancer**, with metastases to his cervical lymph nodes and lungs. He refused conventional chemotherapy and radiation therapy, and opted instead to seek alternative therapy at the Century Wellness Clinic. His chemosensitivity testing showed that certain chemotherapy agents and appropriate supplements would be beneficial in his treatment. This patient has been on low-dose insulin potentiated chemotherapy for the past eighteen months and has had stabilization of his disease, without progression. He has a 100% performance status.

CASE #34—R.K.

A forty-eight-year-old white male dentist from Wisconsin, who was diagnosed with **metastatic gastric cancer** two years ago. He refused conventional chemotherapy. He underwent chemosensitivity testing and was subsequently placed on the FIT protocol. After appropriate chemotherapy agents and appropriate supplements were determined through genetic decoding, the patient returned to the Midwest for follow-up low-dose insulin potentiated therapy at a cancer clinic in Illinois. He continues to practice dentistry and his performance status is 90%.

CASE #35—K.H.

This forty-five-year-old white female from Indiana with **Stage IV breast cancer**, with a proven diagnosis of both lung and bone metastases, decided against full-dose chemotherapy. She was seen at the Century Wellness Clinic for the FIT protocol and for chemosensitivity testing. She was given IV immune therapy and appropriate supplements. When her chemosensitivity test results returned for both appropriate chemotherapy and for appropriate supplements, she embarked on this program, and for the past eighteen months she has been in excellent, full remission with a 100% performance status.

CASE #36—M.P.

This forty-three-year-old white female from Oregon was diagnosed with a large **right breast carcinoma** with bone metastases. She decided against radiation and chemotherapy and was seen at the Century Wellness Clinic, where she underwent chemosensitivity testing. She elected to go on supplements alone with hormonal therapy. After eighteen months she remains in excellent remission with a 100% performance status. She has not experienced any adverse toxicities with the natural therapies.

CASE #37—J.P.

This fifty-six-year-old white male was diagnosed two-and-a-half years ago with a **mesothelioma of the chest**, with involvement of the mediastinum and bilateral pulmonary metastases. This patient rejected full-dose chemotherapy and elected instead to opt for alternative treatments. For the past twenty months he has been in excellent remission and enjoys a 100% performance status. He has not had any adverse toxicities with these natural therapies.

CASE #38—A.D.

This sixty-nine-year-old white male from California was diagnosed with **Stage IV prostate cancer** with bone metastases. He refused radiation therapy, radical prostate surgery, hormonal therapy, and chemotherapy. He sought consultation at the Century Wellness Clinic, where he was placed on the FIT protocol and underwent chemosensitivity testing for determination of the appropriate chemotherapy drugs and appropriate supplements. He is now receiving low-dose insulin potentiated therapy and is enjoying complete remission with a normal PSA level and without any bone pain whatsoever. He has not had any adverse toxicities to any of the treatments thus far.

CASE #39—D.F.

This forty-six-year-old white female from California was diagnosed with **Stage IV breast cancer** with liver metastases. She refused conventional full-dose chemotherapy and opted for alternative therapy instead. After coming to the Century Wellness Clinic she underwent chemosensitivity testing, which determined the appropriate chemotherapy agents, along with the appropriate supplements. Since being on these therapies, along with the FIT protocol, the patient has also started undergoing low-dose insulin potentiated therapy at another clinic closer to her home. She is in excellent remission, presently eighteen months post-initiation of integrative oncology treatment.

CASE #40—C.S.

This seventy-three-year-old white male from Georgia was diagnosed with **Stage IV prostate cancer**, with pelvic and bony metastases. He refused conventional hormonal therapy and did not accept any radiation therapy. The patient underwent chemosensitivity testing, which determined the most suitable drugs and supplements to best treat his metastatic disease, based upon genetic decoding. Following appropriate therapies with insulin potentiation, the patient has had normalization of his PSA levels and he is currently asymptomatic from any bone pain whatsoever. His performance status is 100% and he has not experienced any toxicities from the alternative treatments.

These forty cases represent only a random sampling of the best outcome results from my five-year, 500-patient study. Outcome results refers to complete remission, partial remission, or stable disease condition. Additionally, for the entire 500-patient study, the overall response rate for all of these Stage IV cancers was 45%. The combination of Poly-MVA and other appropriate supplements alone, without any chemotherapy, produced a response rate of 39%, far beyond rates recorded by conventional therapies.

CHAPTER THIRTEEN

FIVE MYTHS ABOUT INTEGRATIVE CANCER TREATMENTS

→ **MYTH #1:** Antioxidants should never be taken by cancer patients because they counteract the effects of radiation therapy and chemotherapy.

→ **FACTS:** You can't find any controlled studies proving this statement to be true because there are no such studies in existence. The myth is perpetuated by conventional oncologists and drug manufacturers based on their fears, not science. When an integrative oncologist prescribes the use of antioxidants, it's intended to bolster the cancer patient's immune system to better deal with both the cancer and any mild side effects caused by low-dose chemo.

→ **MYTH #2:** We all get enough vitamins in a well-balanced diet that extra vitamin supplementation is unnecessary for cancer patients.

→ **FACTS:** When it comes to treating cancer, the guidelines for required daily allowances of vitamins and minerals are worthless. Due to prevailing farming methods and their reliance on chemicals that deplete vitamins and minerals in crops, the average diet is deficient in many important nutrient categories. To counteract these deficiencies, administering high doses of vitamins A, C, E, and D now constitutes the norm among integrative oncologists. Vitamin A in doses of 50,000 to 100,000 IU, for example, has successfully treated head and neck cancers for chemo prevention.

→ **MYTH #3:** The use of various herbal preparations is dangerous and has not been found to be of any value in treating cancer.

→ **FACTS:** High-tech laboratories in Europe and elsewhere that do genetic chemosensitivity testing also routinely test several dozen herbs known among alternative practitioners to be beneficial to cancer patients. Some of these include—E-Tea, quercetin, laetrile, curcumin, pau d'arco, milk thistle, and ukrain. They have no proven record of dangers.

→ **MYTH #4:** There is no treatment value for cancer patients in taking mineral supplements.

→ **FACTS:** Calcium, selenium, zinc, and iodine, to name just a few, are some of the important minerals that are now being acknowledged in the medical literature as having a beneficial effect in the treatment of cancer patients. Conventional oncology is finally beginning to catch up to integrative oncology on this supplementation practice.

→ **MYTH #5:** If alternative and integrative cancer treatments are so effective, my conventional oncologist would have told me or used them him- or herself.

→ **FACTS:** This is the most common myth of all. As I point out in the introduction to this book, most conventional oncologists never learned anything about integrative and alternative cancer treatments in their medical school training. The opportunity to learn has, however, changed in just the last few years, as more than half of all medical schools offer some elective course in alternative medicine.

Another disincentive for conventional oncologists to discuss alternative treatment comes from the Veterans Health Administration hospital system, HMOs, and PPOs, all of which discourage if not forbid their associated physicians from offering or recommending alternatives to strict, high-dose chemotherapy. State medical board regulations also limit the ability of physicians to use any treatments considered to be outside the scope of standard practice.

CHAPTER FOURTEEN

THE CHOICE IS YOURS

Some of the messages and important points that I have made in this book deserve further emphasis.

First, when cancer shows up, as it will in one out of every two men during their lifetime, and in two out of five women during their lifetime, it has probably been developing sub-clinically below the threshold of your awareness for months to years and, yes, you as a patient do have time to make an intelligent and informed decision regarding your treatment. Don't be rushed into feeling that you must make a choice from a limited range of options.

Second, there are a wide variety of treatment options available. Don't let anyone try to convince you differently. Many of these options are "out of the box" of mainstream oncology, and most nontraditional treatments are not covered by state, federal, HMO, or private insurance plans.

However, even some conventional therapies are not allowed or paid for by insurance companies unless the drugs selected are on a list of approved drugs for that particular cancer. This is true even if the chemosensitivity testing shows that certain drugs are effective for a particular individual's cancer and others are not. The review boards of Medicare and private insurance companies have the final say-so.

This amounts to the rationing of care. This practice is already in play in many countries with a socialized medical system. For instance, in Canada and England targeted drugs such as Avastin and Erbitux are too expensive for the system to bear and are just not available to doctors who may order them.

You as a patient have options, and you should exercise those options!

The first option is straight, by-the-book protocol chemotherapy. The next and frequently used option is fractionated low-dose chemotherapy, or the alternative insulin potentiated therapy. The final option is usually complementary treatment alone, or in some integrative (combination) form.

Third, my plea to you as patients is to choose hope and life! Don't allow yourself to be burdened with negativity from oncologists whose only agenda is to get you under the knife, under the radiation beam, or under the IV bottle dripping toxic and often useless chemotherapy.

Your conventional oncologist doesn't possess a crystal ball. If he or she sits behind a desk and gives you an exact time frame as to how long you will remain alive, and talks about hospice care, it is then time to seek out as many alternative treatments as possible.

Base your decision about care on the tools available, especially the high-tech, scientifically based chemosensitivity tests. Chemosensitivity testing gives you the most accurate road map based upon your specific cancer genes and, as much as any other factor, guarantees you a successful outcome as well as the best supplements to aid in your recovery.

Fourth, please never forget that you and every other cancer patient are different from the next, even with the same diagnosis. Your genetic markers are different. Your past medical history is different. Your immune function is different. And, your emotional health is different. A cookie-cutter approach to treating all cancer patients the same, as fostered by Medicare, Medicaid, HMOs, and most private insurance companies, just doesn't work.

Fifth, treatments and changes in protocols should be the rule and not the exception. Keep in mind that a cancer cell is like a smart bacterial infection, as it will almost always find a way to become resistant to certain treatments and to mutate around certain drugs. But these renegade cells can be outsmarted using the multiple tools available to the practice of integrative oncology.

SIX IMPORTANT THINGS TO KEEP IN MIND

Integrative oncologists typically describe for patients these six connections between health and cancer, but rarely if ever will this important information be mentioned to patients by conventional oncologists:

1. Simple-sugar elimination diets are essential to adopt and maintain, as this single act by the patient can deprive the cancer of its main form of nutrition.

2. The best anti-cancer vitamins, minerals, herbs, and amino acids are essential and can be predicted by chemosensitivity testing.

3. The importance of body conditioning, exercise, yoga, Pilates, prayer, and meditation cannot be overemphasized. Keep yourself physically and spiritually healthy!

4. The importance of reducing stress and ridding the mind of toxic emotions, including hate, anger, fear, retribution, and depression, are extremely important.

5. Detoxification of the body from chemical toxins and heavy-metal toxins, including dental amalgams and dental infections, along with colonic cleansing, is an important part of giving the immune system a healthy basis from which to fight any disease.

6. Hormonal balancing with preferably bio-identical hormone replacement therapies, except where contraindicated, can be extremely important in strengthening the immune system and the neuro-endocrine system.

PLACE MORE EMPHASIS ON PREVENTION

We practitioners of integrative oncology place much more emphasis on cancer prevention education than conventional oncologists do because not only do we seek to treat cancer effectively, we want to prevent its recurrence and most importantly, eradicate it from the entire human experience.

For a healthier life free of cancer, we need to think about

what each of us can do to avoid the habits and behaviors that trigger cancer, since the economic burden caused by this disease, and the health-care rationing produced by its occurrence, will only become worse as the years progress.

Imagine how much better you would feel if you would adhere to a healthy, mainly vegetarian diet that is low in red meats, fat, dairy, and fried foods.

Think of how much more energy and stamina you would have if you kept your weight within eight to ten pounds of your ideal body mass index.

By following not only these simple suggestions, but all of the recommendations from the list below, you can significantly decrease your chance of ever developing cancer:

1. Consume lots of fruits, vegetables, and whole grains, preferably organic.
2. Drink bottled and filtered water, preferably alkaline water.
3. Stay away from smoking and smokeless tobacco, and also avoid restaurants, hotels, theaters, and any other enclosed spaces where smokers congregate, in order to avoid passive smoke inhalation.
4. Avoid toxic fumes from gas stations and automobile garages.
5. Avoid living under or near power lines.
6. Avoid houses with high radon levels in the crawl spaces or in the surrounding grounds.
7. Do not engage in risky sexual behavior.
8. Avoid excessive exposure to ultraviolet radiation. Cover your head, arms, and legs with clothing or a sunscreen that has a UVA/UVB protection rating of 30 or higher.

9. Avoid overexposure to microwave and electromagnetic radiation fields.

10. Avoid tanning salons or sunbathing.

11. Take appropriate supplements. (See earlier chapters and appendices for advice.)

12. Avoid excessive radiologic procedures, including CT and PET scans.

13. Take care of your teeth. Floss and have them professionally cleaned often, three or four times per year, and remove old silver fillings and replace with porcelain or composite.

14. Avoid highly toxic, full-dose chemotherapy whenever possible. If a patient is given low-dose insulin potentiated chemotherapy after high-tech chemosensitivity testing identifies the exact drugs, hormones, and supplements best for that particular patient, the cost of treating cancer would be reduced by at least 80% to 90%, which would have positive repercussions for our entire health-care system. The toxic effects of chemotherapy and radiation therapy would either be minimized or completely eliminated. The patient's quality of life would be enhanced tremendously.

All of these goals and lifestyle choices are supported by—and achievable through—the discipline of integrative oncology.

The choice is yours!

THE CANCER PATIENT'S "BILL OF RIGHTS"

1. Right to a positive attitude: Avoid becoming afraid or discouraged, while always knowing that cures for all types of cancers have been reported in the medical literature at one time or another.

2. Freedom to choose an alternate path: Choose an alternative oncologist capable of treating your entire body with the best available pharmaceutical treatments specifically suited to your needs through chemosensitivity testing.

3. Right to remain skeptical: Remain skeptical when reading or hearing statements regarding clinical studies and prognostic results. Always remember that evidence-based medicine is not at play when more than two drugs are used.

4. Right to keep fighting: Politely leave your oncologist's office if he or she starts mentioning "hospice care" or "getting your affairs in order." This means your physician has given up on you, something that no doctor should ever do.

5. Right to change your nutritional habits: Take charge of your diet and nutrition. Be serious about following your medical-support team's dietary recommendations, especially regarding low simple sugars and alkaline recommendations given by naturopathic physicians.

6. Right to say no: Refuse to accept over-testing that involves heavy radiation procedures, especially CT and PET scans, likely to suppress your immune system. Such procedures will prevent your body's immune defenses from working at their optimal levels.

7. Freedom to choose supplements: Always remain aware that there are at least fifty beneficial supplements proven to be helpful in fighting your cancer. Your integrative oncologist should be able to provide results from chemosensitivity testing as to how well specific types of natural substances will assist you.

8. Freedom to question the media: Don't be fooled by advertisements or promotions that claim individual cancer centers have pinpointed radiology procedures. Treatments for specific types of cancer are always localized therapies and the golden rule is that systemic treatments are mandatory for Stage IV cancers.

9. Right to refuse needless surgeries: Avoid yielding to aggressive, life-threatening surgical procedures when your cancer is in Stage IV. Remember, you cannot chase Stage IV disease with a scalpel!

10. Freedom to control your dosage: Whenever possible, use the lowest number of drugs and always use the lowest dose possible to fight your cancer, to prevent destruction and suppression of your immune system.

COMMON CONVENTIONAL TREATMENTS FOR MAJOR CANCERS

I. Breast cancer
    A. Adjuvant therapies:
        i. Adriamycin and Cytoxan followed by Taxol or
           Taxotere (AC+T) every 21 days
        ii. Cytoxan/methotrexate/5-FU (CMF), on day 1 and
           day 8 every 28 days
    B. Stage IV breast cancers:
        i. Cytoxan/Adriamycin/5-FU (FAC) every 21 days
        ii. Taxol/carboplatin, every 28 days
        iii. Velban/Mitomycin-C, every 28 days

II. Colorectal cancer, Stage IV
    A. oxaliplatin/5-FU/leucovorin (Folfox), every 14 days
    B. CPT-11/5-FU/leucovorin (Folfiri), every 14 days
    C. Xeloda (orally)/oxaliplatin (Xelox), every 14 days

III. Esophageal carcinoma, Stage IV
- A. 5-FU/Adriamycin/cisplatin (FAP), every 28 days
- B. Taxol/cisplatin/5-FU, every 28 days
- C. Xeloda (orally)/carboplatin, every 3 weeks

IV. Gastric carcinoma, Stage IV
- A. VP-16/Adriamycin/cisplatin (EAP), every 21 days
- B. VP-16/5-FU/cisplatin (EFP), every 28 days
- C. CPT-11/carboplatin, every 28 days

V. Bladder carcinoma, Stage IV
- A. methotrexate/Velban/Adriamycin/cisplatin (MVAC), every 28 days
- B. Taxotere/carboplatin, every 21 days
- C. Carboplatin/Gemzar, every 28 days

VI. Prostate carcinoma, Stage IV (hormone independent)
- A. Taxotere, weekly, 3 out of 4 weeks per month
- B. mitoxantrone/prednisone, every 21 days
- C. VP-16/estramustine (orally), every 28 days

VII. Renal cell carcinoma, Stage IV
- A. Nexavar (orally)
- B. Sutent (orally)
- C. alpha interferon-2a/interleukin-2

VIII. Testicular carcinoma, Stage IV
- A. cisplatin/bleomycin/VP-16 (BEP), every 21 days
- B. Taxol/Gemzar, every 28 days
- C. Velban/Ifex/cisplatin/mesna, every 21 days

IX. Cervical carcinoma, Stage IV
- A. bleomycin/Ifex/cisplatin, every 21 days

B. Taxol/carboplatin, every 21 days

C. methotrexate/Velban/Adriamycin/cisplatin, every 28 days

X. Endometrial (uterine) carcinoma, Stage IV

  A. cisplatin/Taxol, every 21 days

  B. cisplatin/Adriamycin/Cytoxan, every 28 days

  C. Taxotere, weekly, 3 out of 4 weeks per month

XI. Ovarian carcinoma, Stage IV

  A. carboplatin/Taxol, every 21 days

  B. Cytoxan/cisplatin, every 21 days

  C. Doxil, every 3 weeks

XII. Head and neck carcinoma, Stage IV

  A. carboplatin/5-FU/Taxol, every 21 days

  B. carboplatin/Taxotere, every 21 days

  C. Navelbine/carboplatin, every 21 days

XIII. Lung carcinoma, Stage IV

  A. Non-small-cell carcinoma (NSC), Stage IV

    i. carboplatin/Taxol, every 21 days

    ii. carboplatin/Navelbine, every 28 days

    iii. carboplatin/Gemzar, every 28 days

  B. Small-cell carcinoma (SCC), Stage IV

    i. Adriamycin/Cytoxan/VP-16, every 21 days

    ii. Cytoxan/Adriamycin/vincristine, every 21 days

    iii. Ifex/mesna/carboplatin/VP-16, every 28 days

XIV. Hodgkin's disease, Stage IV

  A. Adriamycin/bleomycin/Velban/DTIC, every 28 days

  B. Mustargen/vincristine/procarbazine/prednisone, every 28 days

C. Adriamycin/Velban/Mustargen/vincristine/
bleomycin/VP-16, every 28 days

XV. Non-Hodgkin's lymphoma (NHL), Stage IV
A. Cytoxan/Adriamycin/vincristine/prednisone/
Rituxan (R-CHOP), every 21 days
B. Cytoxan/vincristine/prednisone (CVP), every 21 days
C. VP-16/prednisone/cytarabine/cisplatin, every
28 days

XVI. Melanoma, Stage IV
A. bleomycin/vincristine/lomustine/dacarbazine,
every 28 days
B. Velban/bleomycin/cisplatin, every 28 days
C. dacarbazine/dactinomycin, every 21 days

XVII. Multiple myeloma, Stage IV
A. Velcade/dexamethasone, every 21 days
B. thalidomide/Cytoxan/VP-16/dexamethasone,
every 28 days
C. melphalan/prednisone, days 1 through 4, every
28 days

XVIII. Primary brain tumors (adult)
A. Temodar, days 1 through 5, every 28 days
B. procarbazine/CCNU/vincristine, every 28 days

XIX. Pancreatic carcinoma, Stage IV
A. Gemzar/5-FU, every week, 3 out of 4 weeks
B. Adriamycin/Mitomycin-C/5-FU, every 28 days
C. Gemzar/Tarceva; Gemzar given weekly via IV,
Tarceva given daily orally

DR. FORSYTHE'S GENERAL CANCER SUPPORT FORMULA

A. Serving size: one packet per day

B. Amount per serving:
   1. Adrenal essence   *
   2. Artemisia complex   *
   3. Astragalus   250 mg
   4. Beta-glucan   200 mg
   5. Colostrum   *
   6. DHEA   25 mg
   7. DIMension 3   150 mg
   8. E-Tea   *
   9. Glyco Essentials   *
   10. Immunotix 3-6   *
   11. IP-6   1000 mg
   12. L-lysine   500 mg
   13. Melatonin   5 mg
   14. Quercetin   300 mg
   15. Resveratrol   125 mg

16. Vitamin C   3000 mg
17. Vitamin D   35000 IU

* Proprietary

DR. FORSYTHE'S BRAIN SUPPORT FORMULA

A. Serving size: one packet daily
B. Amount per serving:
    1. Acetyl-carnitine   200 mg
    2. Alpha-lipoic acid   200 mg
    3. Astragalus   250 mg
    4. Vitamin B-complex   *
    5. Choline   100 mcg
    6. Folic acid   400 mcg
    7. Ginkgo extract   135 mcg
    8. Glutathione   5 mg
    9. Glyco Essentials   *
    10. Grape-seed extract   5 mg
    11. IP-6   1020 mg
    12. Melatonin   5 mg
    13. Milk thistle extract   25 mg
    14. N-Acetylcysteine   350 mg
    15. Quercetin   300 mg
    16. Resveratrol   125 mg
    17. Selenium   200 mcg
    18. Vitamin C   3000 mg
    19. Vitamin D   35000 IU
    20. Vitamin E   800 IU
    21. Zinc   25 mg

* Proprietary

DR. FORSYTHE'S BREAST SUPPORT FORMULA

A. Supplemental facts - serving size: one packet daily
B. Amount per serving:

1.	Alpha-lipoic acid	200 mg
2.	Astragalus	250 mg
3.	Vitamin B-complex	*
4.	Beta-carotene	30,000 IU
5.	Beta-glucan	200 mg
6.	Calcium	1000 mg
7.	CoQ-10	300 mg
8.	Cordyceps	27 mg
9.	DIMension 3	*
10.	E-Tea	*
11.	Folate	400 mcg
12.	Glutathione	5 mg
13.	Glyco Essentials	*
14.	Iodine	150 mcg
15.	IP-6	1020 mg
16.	Mushroom extract	27 mg
17.	Milk thistle	25 mg
18.	N-Acetylcysteine	50 mg
19.	Quercetin	300 mg
20.	Resveratrol	125 mg
21.	Selenium	200 mcg
22.	Vitamin C	3000 mg
23.	Vitamin D	35000 IU
24.	Vitamin E	400 IU
25.	Zinc	25 mg

* Proprietary

DR. FORSYTHE'S COLORECTAL SUPPORT FORMULA

A. Supplemental facts - serving size: onc packet daily
B. Amount per serving:
    1. Aloe vera extract   250 mg
    2. Alpha-lipoic acid   200 mg
    3. Vitamin B-Complex   *
    4. Beta-carotene   30,000 IU
    5. Calcium   1000 mg
    6. Citrus bioflavonoid complex   *
    7. Glutathione   5 mg
    8. Glyco Essentials   *
    9. Lutein   9 mcg
   10. Melatonin   5 mg
   11. Milk thistle extract   95 mg
   12. Pancreatin   200 mg
   13. Pau-d'arco   100 mg
   14. Pro-Bio Defense   *
   15. Quercetin   300 mg
   16. Resveratrol   125 mg
   17. Selenium   200 mcg
   18. Turmeric extract   6 mg
   19. Vitamin C   3000 mg
   20. Vitamin D   35000 IU
   21. Vitamin E   400 IU
   22. Zinc   25 mg

* Proprietary

DR. FORSYTHE'S LYMPHOMA SUPPORT FORMULA

A.   Supplemental facts - serving size: one packet daily

B.   Amount per serving:

1.	Adrenal essence	*
2.	Alpha-lipoic acid	200 mg
3.	Beta-glucan	200 mg
4.	Calcium	1000 mg
5.	Citrus bioflavonoid complex	250 mg
6.	CoQ-10	300 mg
7.	Colostrum	*
8.	Cordyceps	27 mg
9.	Folate	400 mcg
10.	Glutathione	5 mg
11.	Glyco Essentials	*
12.	Grape-seed extract	5 mg
13.	Iodine	150 mcg
14.	IP-6	1020 mg
15.	Magnesium	500 mg
16.	Milk thistle extract	95 mg
17.	Mushroom extract	*
18.	Olive leaf extract	400 mg
19.	Quercetin	300 mg
20.	Resveratrol	125 mg
21.	Selenium	200 mcg
22.	Vitamin C	3000 mg
23.	Vitamin D	35000 IU
24.	Vitamin E	400 IU
25.	Zinc	25 mg

* Proprietary

DR. FORSYTHE'S LUNG SUPPORT FORMULA

A. Supplemental facts - serving size: one packet daily
B. Amount per serving:
   1. Alpha-lipoic acid   400 mg
   2. Astragalus   250 mg
   3. Vitamin B-Complex   *
   4. Beta-glucan   200 mg
   5. Calcium   1000 mg
   6. Citrus bioflavonoid complex   100 mg
   7. CoQ-10   300 mg
   8. Colostrum   *
   9. Cordyceps   27 mg
   10. E-Tea   *
   11. Folate   400 mcg
   12. Glutathione   5 mg
   13. Glyco Essentials   *
   14. Grape-seed extract   5 mg
   15. Green tea extract   *
   16. Iodine   150 mcg
   17. L-lysine   500 mg
   18. Magnesium   500 mg
   19. Milk thistle extract   25 mg
   20. Mushroom extract   *
   21. Quercetin   300 mg
   22. Resveratrol   125 mg
   23. Selenium   200 mcg
   24. Turmeric extract   6 mg
   25. Vitamin C   3000 mg
   26. Vitamin D3   5000 IU
   27. Vitamin E   400 IU
   28. Zinc   25 mg

* Proprietary

DR. FORSYTHE'S OVARIAN SUPPORT FORMULA

A. Supplemental facts - serving size: one packet daily
B. Amount per serving:
    1. Alpha-lipoic acid   200 mg
    2. Astragalus   250 mg
    3. Vitamin B-Complex   *
    4. Beta-glucan   200 mg
    5. Calcium   1000 mg
    6. Citrus bioflavonoid complex   250 mg
    7. CoQ-10   300 mg
    8. Colostrum   27 mg
    9. Cordyceps   27 mg
    10. DIMension 3   150 mg
    11. Folate   400 mcg
    12. Glutathione   5 mg
    13. Glyco Essentials   *
    14. Grape-seed extract   55 mg
    15. Iodine   150 mcg
    16. Magnesium   500 mg
    17. Milk thistle extract   25 mg
    18. Mushroom extract   *
    19. Olive leaf extract   400 mg
    20. Quercetin   300 mg
    21. Resveratrol   125 mg
    22. Selenium   200 mcg
    23. Turmeric extract   6 mg
    24. Vitamin A   3000 IU
    25. Vitamin C   3000 mg
    26. Vitamin D   35000 IU
    27. Vitamin E   400 IU
    28. Zinc   25 mg

* Proprietary

DR. FORSYTHE'S PROSTATE SUPPORT FORMULA

A. Supplemental facts - serving size: one packet daily

B. Amount per serving:

1.	Alpha-lipoic acid	200 mg
2.	Astragalus	500 mg
3.	Vitamin B-Complex	*
4.	Calcium	1000 mg
5.	Calcium D-glucarate	200 mg
6.	Citrus bioflavonoid complex	*
7.	CoQ-10	300 mg
8.	Folate	400 mcg
9.	Glutathione	5 mg
10.	Glyco Essentials	*
11.	Grape-seed extract	*
12.	Iodine	150 mcg
13.	DIMension 3	*
14.	IP-6	800 mg
15.	Lutein	36 mcg
16.	Lycopene	2.5 mg
17.	Magnesium	500 mg
18.	Mushroom extract	*
19.	Melatonin	5 mg
20.	Milk thistle extract	25 mg
21.	Modified citrus pectin	2000 mg
22.	ProstaFlo	*
23.	Quercetin	300 mg
24.	Resveratrol	125 mg
25.	Saw palmetto	160 mg
26.	Selenium	200 mcg
27.	Vitamin A	30,000 IU
28.	Vitamin C	3000 mg

29. Vitamin D   35000 IU
30. Vitamin E   400 IU
31. Zinc   25 mg

* Proprietary

INTEGRATIVE CANCER TREATMENT RESOURCES

The following organizations and Web sites are of value in finding doctors, homeopaths, and naturopaths in your area to guide you in your search for optimal treatment outcomes:

American Academy of Anti-Aging Medicine (A4M)
1510 West Montana Street, Chicago, IL 60614
(773) 528-4333
www.worldhealth.net

American College for Advancement in Medicine
(ACAM)
23121 Verdugo Drive, Suite 204, Laguna Hills, CA
  92653
(800) 532-3688
www.acamnet.org

Cancer Control Society
2043 North Berendo Street, Los Angeles, CA 90027
(323) 663-7801
www.cancercontrolsociety.com

LifeExtension Foundation
5990 North Federal Highway, Fort Lauderdale, FL
    33308
(800) 226-2370
www.lef.org

The Best Answer for Cancer Foundation
8127 Mesa, b-206, #243, Austin, TX 78759
(512) 342-8181
www.bestanswerforcancer.org

The contact information for the important chemosensitivity testing international laboratories include:

Biofocus Institute for Laboratory Medicine
Dr. Doris Bachg and Dr. Uwe Haselhorst
    (Pathologists)
Berghäuser Strasse 295, 45659 Recklinghausen,
    Germany
Contact: Dr. L. Prix
+49-2361-3000-130
www.biofocus.de/
e-mail: prix@biofocus.de

Research Genetic Cancer Centre (RGCC)
PO Box 53070, Florina, Greece

+30-24630-42264

email: jpapasot@doctors.org.uk

Dr. Ray Hammon

6822 22nd Avenue, North #332, St. Petersburg, FL
    33710

(727) 345-2050

www.rgccusa.com

info@rgccusa.com

Goodgene Molecular Genetic Testing Center

11F, Mario Digital Tower, 222-12, Gurodong, Guro-
    Gu, Seoul 150-050, South Korea

PH: +82-2-3409-0561

FAX: +82-2-6218-0562

www.goodgene.co.kr

TESTING FOR TOXINS AND NUTRITIONAL DEFICIENCIES:

Doctor's Data, Inc.

3755 Illinois Avenue, St. Charles, IL 60174

(800) 323-2784

For outside the US and Canada: (630) 377-8139

www.doctorsdata.com

SELECTED IPT/IPTLD PHYSICIANS:

- **ALASKA**

  Anchorage

  Michael J. Ellenburg, ND

  3500 Latouche Street, Anchorage AK 99518

  (907) 563-2366

  www.drellenburg.com

- **ARIZONA**

  David Korn, MD, DO, DDS

  LongLife Medical, Inc.

  6632 East Baseline Road, Suite 105, Mesa, AZ
     85206

  (480) 354-6700

  www.longlife-medical.com

  Thomas Lodi, MD

  An Oasis of Healing

  210 North Center Street, Suite 102, Mesa, AZ
     85201

  (480) 834-5414

  www.anoasisofhealing.com

  Charles Schwengel, DO

  Medicine of HOPE

  4550 East Bell Road, Suite 284, Phoenix,
     AZ 85032

  (877) 668-1448

  Medicineofhope.com

- **CALIFORNIA**

  Oceanside

  Les Breitman, MD

  Juergen Winkler, MD

  Alternative Cancer Treatment Center of
      Southern California

  2204 El Camino Real, Suite 104, Oceanside,
      CA 92054

  (760) 439-9955

  www.ipthealing.com

  Santa Rosa

  Robert J. Rowen, MD

  PO Box 817, Santa Rosa, CA 95403

  (707) 578-7787

  www.secondopinionnewsletter.com

- **FLORIDA**

  Sunny Isles

  Martin Dayton, DO

  Dayton Medical Center, 18600 Collins Avenue,
      Sunny Isles Beach, FL 33160

  (305) 931-8484

  www.daytonmedical.com

- **ILLINOIS**

  Burr Ridge

  Steven Ayre, MD

  Ather Malik, DO

  Contemporary Medicine, 322 Burr Ridge
      Parkway, Burr Ridge, IL 60527

(630) 321-9010

www.contemporarymedicine.net

- **INDIANA**

  Indianapolis

  Dale Guyer, MD

  Advanced Medical Center and Spa, 836 East 86th
      Street, Indianapolis, IN 46240

  (317) 580-9355

  www.daleguyermd.com

- **MICHIGAN**

  Ann Arbor

  Thomas Kabisch, DO

  2330 East Stadium, Suite 2, Ann Arbor, MI 48104

  (734) 971-5483

- **NEW MEXICO**

  Santa Fe

  Hennie Fitzpatrick, MD

  Integrative Health Medical Center, 1532-A Cer-
      rillos Road, Sante Fe, NM 87505

  (505) 982-3936

  www.drhennie.com

- **NEVADA**

  Carson City

  Frank Shallenberger, MD, HMD

  The Nevada Center of Alternative & Anti-Aging
      Medicine, 1231 Country Club Drive, Carson
      City, NV 89703

(775) 884-3990

www.antiagingmedicine.com

Reno

James W. Forsythe, MD, HMD

Century Wellness Clinic, 521 Hammill Lane,
    Reno, NV 89511

(775) 827-0707 or (877) 789-0707

www.drforsythe.com

· **NEW YORK**

Glen Cove/Long Island

Richard Linchitz, MD

Linchitz Medical Wellness, PLLC, 70 Glen Street,
    Suite 240, Glen Cove, NY 11542

(516) 759-4200

http://linchitzwellness.com

· **OHIO**

Mansfield

Juan Penhos, MD

Get Well Center, 635 South Trimble Road, Mans-
    field, OH 44906

(419) 524-2676

http://allgetwell.com

· **TEXAS**

Dallas

Constantine Kotsanis, MD

The Kotsanis Institute, 2020 West Highway 114,
    Suite 260, Grapevine, TX 76051

(817) 380-4992 or (888) 302-9740

www.kotsanisinstitute.com

- **WASHINGTON**

Seattle

Brad Weeks, MD

The Weeks Clinic for Corrective Medicine and
Psychiatry

6456 South Central Avenue, PO Box 740,
Clinton, WA 98236

PH: (360) 341-2303

FAX: (360) 341-2313

http://weeksmd.com

ACKNOWLEDGMENTS

To my entire office staff for their encouragement and dedication, and to my talented transcriptionist, Diane Comstock. To the publishing genius Bill Gladstone of Waterside Productions and his amazing editor and ghostwriter Randall Fitzgerald, whose talents are, in a word, *Excelsior.*

To our public relations director, Patty Melton, her husband, Wayne Melton, and her partner, Margie Enlow, whose expertise and creativity in putting this entire package together are much appreciated.

To my friend, mentor, and longtime supporter, Dr. Burton Goldberg, for writing the foreword and who, for the past twenty years, has expressed his beliefs in several dozen books and articles for improving integrative cancer therapies through his worldwide travels and research. His expertise and research have been instrumental in introducing me to the use of high-tech chemosensitivity testing in order to "blueprint" the best drugs and the best supplements that allow a specific protocol for each individual patient, which is then preferably followed with low-dose insulin potentiated therapy.

BIBLIOGRAPHY

The majority of information in this book comes from the author's many years of practicing oncology, reading and contributing to medical journals, attending conferences, and his ongoing education. The facts and figures in this book have been taken from the following locations:

Morgan, Graeme et al. "The Contribution of Cytotoxic Chemotherapy to 5-year Survival in Adult Malignancies." *Clinical Oncology* (2004) 16: 549–560.

American Cancer Society, www.cancer.org

US Public Health Service, www.usphs.gov

World Health Organization, www.who.int/en/

INDEX